# Teaching and Assessing Nurses

# Teaching and Assessing Nurses

## A Handbook for Preceptors

**ROBERT OLIVER**

and

**COLIN ENDERSBY**

*Baillière Tindall*

LONDON • PHILADELPHIA • TORONTO • SYDNEY • TOKYO

*Baillière Tindall*   24-28 Oval Road
W. B. Saunders   London NW1 7DX

The Curtis Center
Independence Square West
Philadelphia, PA 19106-3399, USA

Harcourt Brace & Company
55 Horner Avenue
Toronto, Ontario, M8Z 4X6, Canada

Harcourt Brace & Company, Australia
30-52 Smidmore Street
Marrickville
NSW 2204, Australia

Harcourt Brace & Company, Japan
Ichibancho Central Building
22-1 Ichibancho
Chiyoda-ku, Tokyo 102, Japan

A catalogue record for this book is available from the British Library

ISBN 0-7020-1720-5

Typeset by Mathematical Composition Setters Ltd, Salisbury, Wiltshire

Printed and bound in Great Britain by the Bath Press, Avon

# Contents

# The Editors

**ROBERT OLIVER**
BSc, RGN, RSCN, Cert Ed (FE), FETC
Associate Lecturer,
Faculty of Health and Social Work,
Anglia Polytechnic University,
Freelance lecturer specialising in
developing and delivering staff
education and development
and author of
*Psychology for Nurses*
also published by
Baillière Tindall

**COLIN ENDERSBY**
RGN, RCNT, Cert Ed (FE)
Associate Lecturer,
Faculty of Health and Social Work,
Anglia Polytechnic University and
Freelance lecturer specialising in
developing and delivering staff
education and development

# Introduction

Any profession which relies on practical experience for students of that profession must at some time address the problems of who is going to teach and assess them, and what preparation will they need in order to be able to do this. Since the mid 1980s the nursing profession has identified a specific course (ENB 997/998, Teaching and Assessing in Clinical Practice) which prepares trained nurses for this role. With the advent of the ENB's Framework and Higher Award the traditional 997/998 courses are likely to be provided by participants undertaking a teaching module and then an assessing module in the future. However, the subjects discussed here remain relevant whichever format is used.

On the surface it would appear that this is the end of the story, i.e. we have nurses who need to learn in the practical situation, therefore you train someone to do it. The problem is not a simple one to solve, and several ongoing themes need to be addressed before the nature of such training becomes effective.

Firstly, there is the problem of teaching in the clinical area and the different teaching strategies that should be employed in order to achieve this. It is not enough to assume that all teaching occurring in the clinical area is by demonstration and all teaching occurring in university is by seminar and lecture. It is not suggested that anybody would assume these oversimplistic facts to be true, but it is an easy trap to fall into to assume that teaching strategies can be categorised in this way. Much of the debate would appear to originate within the areas of deciding what exactly is to be achieved in both the academic and clinical setting, and the assumptions underlying this text are that although there are important differences, there is nevertheless a great deal of overlap.

The point is made throughout the text that students should be encouraged to formulate their own learning outcomes or at least be able to define their own starting point when approaching a subject and this may necessitate the use of some teacher-centred approaches and may even encroach (indeed should) on the academic classroom-based learning that the student has already undergone.

Secondly, there is the nature of the students themselves to consider. With the advent of Project 2000, the term "supernumerary status" has become well known to all of us, but less well known are the meanings that underlie it. It does not mean standing and watching all the time without ever becoming involved, neither does it mean remaining outside the clinical situation. The assumptions made in this text are that the student should become a part of the clinical team and should feel as though their contributions are worthwhile.

Thirdly, the classic debate of whether the student's course of study is product or process based is still raging between those involved in the education of students. It cannot be denied that the object of nurse education is to facilitate a practitioner with defined competences and hence is, to an extent, product based. This text, in accepting this fact places great emphasis on the process of education and some of the psychological considerations connected with it.

Like any other textbook this one has a rationale behind not only its organisation, but also its style. The arrangement of chapters is such that it takes the reader initially through communication and learning which the individual will need not only for their own use but also in order to guide others. Towards the end of the text the emphasis is placed on the nurse in the clinical area as being a part of the education team in such areas as curriculum planning.

The first part of the text deals with factors which affect teaching and learning of basic skills, and which are essential to both. It is hoped that by dissecting subjects such as communication, attitudes, memory, perception and motivation, that a greater understanding of the learning process will ensue.

Planning a learning experience along with designing the resources to facilitate it and maintaining a learning environment conducive to it are seen as central focuses of the teaching role of the clinical nurse. Included in these chapters are items such as auditing and quality assurance, which will contribute to the overall nature of the learning environment, which uses as its basis the assumption that all must be involved in these processes.

The assessment of students is covered not only from the point of view of the practicalities involved, but also from the planning viewpoint. It is hoped that using this approach will facilitate a greater understanding of the construction and use of the assessment strategies, and will foster more critical analysis of systems used. Similarly, the curriculum planning section is in more detail than is traditionally given in texts written for the ENB 998 course, but at the same time, as throughout the rest of the text, practical guidelines are given which should make participation in the curriculum planning process more rewarding.

Finally, study skills are discussed; these are seen as an essential part of any course. Appendices are provided on such things as how to carry out a literature search and writing references, to complete this subject.

The textbook is written from the viewpoint that the nurse involved in teaching in the clinical area has an importance equal to the other members of the education team, and as such, extensive references are given which will enable the reader to look in more depth at the subject and to participate fully in the process.

The inclusion of activities at the end of each chapter is to enhance the content of the textbook, in many cases through the experience of talking to others constructively, and investigating current practice. They have emerged as a result of extensive use and modification by the authors, in teaching the ENB 998 course.

chapter one

# Communication

## Introduction

Communicating with other individuals appears to be such a basic function that its various ramifications are easy to overlook. Its importance in all spheres of health care has been highlighted by numerous authors, particularly in terms of the consequences in the event of communication breakdown (e.g. Ley, 1982).

The importance of effective communication in the learning environment requires no less attention, but instead of just presenting an account of how communication can be improved we should firstly look at some of the more important factors that contribute to this nebulous subject, and to consider why the message that is given by one person is not necessarily being effectively picked up by others. The subject of communication will be revisited in more specific terms throughout the rest of the text.

In looking at communication, both the verbal and non-verbal aspects will be briefly explored.

## Non-verbal communication

During any face-to-face encounter, the type of body language exhibited can make a difference to how a message is interpreted, sometimes regardless of the words that are actually used. To consider any one behaviour in isolation without placing it within a wider context of behaviour would be wrong (Kendon, 1982), as even silence and immobility can be important in an interaction (Attwell, 1974). Care must therefore be taken with interpreting "hidden meanings" to messages based on isolated behaviours, such as avoiding eye contact. Non-verbal behaviour carries information about, and can even regulate, the immediate social situation.

Probably the most useful classification of non-verbal behaviours is that proposed by Ekman and Friesen (1969). With this classification, it is assumed that non-verbal signs have various functions:

*Emblems* – signs which are complete in themselves, e.g. the "thumbs-up" sign.
*Illustrators* – signs which supplement speech, e.g. pointing whilst giving directions.
*Regulators* – behaviours which control the interaction, e.g. using eye contact to control a conversation.
*Affect displays* – the expression of emotion, e.g. by facial expression.
*Adaptors* – attempts to maintain self-control, e.g. fidgeting.

Research has shown repeatedly (e.g. Morris, 1977) that we say things with our bodies that we neither intend to say nor are aware of saying. *Non-verbal leakage* is the process of physical responses which are conveying a different message to the words being used at the time. In other words when people tell lies, the trained observer can recognise the fact by watching their body language. For most of us, we are often left with, perhaps a feeling of uneasiness following an encounter as we have detected cues, probably unconsciously, which do not match what was said.

In terms of how we may impart information non-verbally, broadly the behaviours fall into the following categories:

1. Facial expressions.
2. Eye contact.
3. Physical Proximity.
4. Physical appearance
5. Posture.
6. Bodily contact.
7. Gestures – involuntary, body orientation, movements.

## Facial expressions

Far from being the easiest non-verbal cue to interpret, facial expressions are probably the most complicated and confusing, and unlike many other non-verbal behaviours, will often continue even if the person is alone (Ekman, 1982). Although one of the prime functions of facial expressions is to communicate emotion (Argyle, 1983), there are times when social interaction can actually dampen down facial expressions of emotion (Ekman, 1972).

Expressions, such as those used to express happiness, anger, sadness, etc., are perhaps the easiest to falsify, particularly over a brief period of time, and indeed to an extent, our society demands that under certain circumstances we should do just that. Meeting people that we do not really wish to see, or being at a social gathering that we would rather avoid, are just two examples where a "mask" of happiness is almost demanded by other people around us.

It makes sense, therefore not to rely solely on the facial expression to provide information about how the individual is reacting, and possibly the most revealing behaviour is not the expression but the mode of eye contact.

## Eye contact

Studies into the significance of different aspects of eye contact have revealed its uses in regulating conversations (Kendon, 1967), when it was found that although speakers would tend to look away from the listener after about five seconds, they would again initiate eye contact when they expected a response. Exline *et al.* (1979), whilst investigating the direction of gaze, found that subjects recounting sad experiences were likely to look down for significant amounts of the interaction.

There is enormous variation between individuals and indeed cultures, and so it is not surprising to reiterate the fact that eye contact alone is not a reliable indicator, and should be considered in connection with other facial expressions and in the context of the interaction.

## Physical proximity and posture

The distance between two people has been found to have an effect on the interaction that takes place, and indeed the situation and relationship of the participants will usually determine this distance in the first place (Hall, 1979). Hall divides these distances broadly into four categories:

Intimate                $0-1\frac{1}{2}$ ft
Casual/personal         $1\frac{1}{2}-4$ ft
Social/consultative     4–12 ft
Public                  12 ft or more

Again, there is tremendous cultural variation in these distances, although the categories remain reasonably constant.

To intrude into a person's intimate space without permission is likely to prompt discomfort at the very least and may even provoke an aggressive response, although conversely too wide a space could be construed as "stand-offish". From a teaching point of view, it has been suggested by at least one author that effective teachers tend to stand closer to the students than do ineffective ones, although the reasons for this are still unclear, and as the author points out, this is a more subjective than objective observation.

Naturally, physical proximity may depend on the postures adopted by the participants (sitting, standing, etc.). The same rules will apply, if possible, when orientating themselves, but may take the form of moving chairs, or even ensuring that a table or desk is placed between the parties with the result that the space is increased. The postures that we adopt may indicate tension, relaxation, interest, or even a desire to be somewhere else! In particular, if we are interested in what a person is saying to us, especially if we like the person, then we may reflect their body movements, and this is called "mirroring". This effect is often seen when individuals are engaged in conversations of mutual interest, and can include such postures as leaning forward, and together with facial expressions, is easy to manipulate.

## Physical appearance

The individual's physical appearance will often lead us to form a first impression about them. They may remind us of someone else, we may compare their manner of dressing with ours, and indeed we may form impressions about what the person is wearing.

This not a particularly accurate way of interpreting body language, not least of all because of the many reasons that may underlie a person's appearance.

## Bodily contact

Face to face interactions will frequently involve bodily contact, and naturally, physical proximity and posture will be important non-verbal indicators in the nature of contact that may occur (Kendon, 1982). In order for bodily contact, including ritualistic behaviours such as handshaking, to be comfortable, both parties should have a common, or at least a complementary goal.

In terms of the ritualistic behaviours, such common goals are often dictated by society, and participants will orientate themselves spatially, maintain eye contact, etc., in order to carry out the action. Bodily contact which is complementary may consist of one person fulfilling another's need for physical comfort following an upsetting experience, by using consoling actions such as touching an arm, holding hands or even cuddling.

In initial contacts with people, particularly when it is expected that the relationship will be fairly long term and that both parties may encounter stress, some form of "channel opening" is a good idea. "Guiding" behaviours such as shoulder touching when the person is leaving, or arm touching as a greeting, may make bodily contact easier to use in times of crisis when more "invasion" (in terms of proximity) may be needed.

# Gestures

Gestures are used worldwide to emphasise points, control conversations and to express emotions. There is, again, needless to say, considerable variation between cultures (Morris, 1977), although there do appear to be some common core gestures which have international meaning. This similarity and difference can lead to confusion as a person from one culture noticing a gesture from another culture may misinterpret it.

*Baton signs* (hand gestures) have been extensively described and range from the "attack" sign of finger pointing (raised forefinger baton) to those which give us information about the content of the message and attitude of the individual such as the finger–thumb touch (hand purse) which indicates precision and a quest for detail. Movements which involve the hands and face in conjunction, such as covering the mouth (doubt), stroking the chin (concentration), rubbing the back of the neck (preoccupation) and eye rubbing (avoiding eye contact) are perhaps the more common ones.

Baton signs utilising the position of the palms are the most easily manipulated in order to convey a message that the conveyor wishes to impart. Palms up indicates begging behaviour in which the individual is seeking acceptance and may be used when trying to introduce controversial topics into a session. Similarly cooperation with other individuals can be sought by the palm side action, which indicates that the individual wishes to bridge a gap. Palm forwards will indicate that the individual wishes the other person not to intervene whereas the palm down will indicate a desire to calm the situation down. Finally, palms pointed towards the individual who is giving the message, may indicate that they are attempting to embrace an idea. Preceptors should be aware that their feelings may be unconsciously conveyed, particularly through these baton signs (non-verbal leakage) and this may cause discomfort in the person receiving the message and should be avoided if possible.

# Listening skills

Certain behaviours indicate that we are listening, and conversely, some may indicate that we are preoccupied or even disinterested. Sitting directly opposite a person can be threatening, particularly if the physical proximity infringes into the intimate space. Sitting at about a ninety-degree angle is usually advisable unless the two parties are very well acquainted. An open posture is advisable in order to indicate that the listener does not feel threatened or preoccupied. Generally, arms and legs being crossed and tucked under do not indicate receptiveness to what is being said.

It has already been discussed that a close relationship is typified by the mirroring of body movements and most obviously the movement of leaning forward to show concern can be used. This does not mean that during the entire encounter the listener needs to be perched on the end of a chair, but rather that it may be used effectively when the other person indicates difficulty in expressing themselves.

The importance and pattern of eye contact has been discussed earlier, and it will be remembered that continuous eye gaze can be threatening, or at least will send out the wrong messages! Intermittent eye contact is preferable.

Finally, the listener should not indicate tension but should rather indicate that they are relaxed and want to listen.

# Communication interference

Interference with the communication process is a common phenomenon, and is frequently termed "noise". The term is rather misleading as it not only refers to noise in the usual sense, but also to any factor, both physical (e.g. discomfort) and psychological (e.g. attitudes), that can adversely affect the passage of a message from one person to another.

The reasons why we do not receive the message as it was intended may, however, be even more simple. Briefly, interference may be caused by quite personal factors:

1. We do not like the communicator.
2. We do not see the relevance of the message.
3. We think that we have something better to say.
4. We are not motivated to listen.
5. We are trying to anticipate what the other person may say.
6. We are thinking about something else.
7. We are prejudiced against the subject.
8. We did not actually hear it.
9. We did not understand the language.

Conversely we may listen to the message because we like or admire the speaker, or we feel that we will need to take action as a result of the message, or there are no other distractions around at the time!

# Encoding and decoding

*Encoding* refers to the process of converting an idea into symbols (words). Conversely, *decoding* is the process by which we translate words back into ideas. In order for communication to be effective between two or more people, the conventions for encoding and decoding need to correspond (Lantz and Stefflre, 1964).

The extent to which conventions are shared by different occupational groups was being investigated as long ago as 1945 (Elkin), although in the context of the groups involved in this text, the picture is slightly different, in as much as the two groups involved (students and trained staff) share a common profession, with the major differences being experience and seniority.

If we take the example of a teaching session given by a senior member of staff to a group of very junior nurses, we can see how such a mechanism can impair the communication process. The "teacher" may mention in the course of a session the term "cardiac failure", which is an encoded term. If the student has no previous knowledge of this phenomenon, and is unable to ask what it is, then they may decode it as "heart attack", "coronary", etc., with the term "failure" leading them to assume that concepts are the same. The conclusions that can be drawn from the above example, relate to altering the conventions in a way that the message which we encode is decoded correctly, and the most effective way of achieving this is by giving full explanations to the student, or more obviously, using language which is within the student's scope of experience.

# Elaborate and restricted codes

Talking in a language that no one can understand is one thing, but often the problem that arises is that the message lacks substance, is over-simplistic and contains no explanation. This is known as a *restricted code*. Educationally, information given in this manner has little or no place, as the student will either carry out instructions wrongly, or will carry them out without any real idea as to why they are doing it. It should not be assumed that the student will ask if they require an explanation, nor that they already understand the meanings behind procedures.

The alternative to the restricted code is the elaborate code, where explanations are given and consequently clarification may be invited from the student.

# Transactional analysis (Berne, 1964)

The way in which information is relayed to another individual has so far been examined in terms of the language we use, our non-verbal behaviours and the ways in which the message is prevented from being received accurately. Berne (1964), in discussing the interactions between individuals, described a "system of feelings accompanied by a set of coherent behaviour patterns". These he termed *ego states*, of which there are three:

Parent;
Adult;
Child;

or in Berne's terminology:

exteropsychic;
neopsychic;
archaeopsychic.

During any interaction we will exhibit one of these ego states, although they are quite fluid and are affected by emotion, attitudes, circumstances, and perhaps most importantly of all, the reaction we are getting from the individual that we are interacting with.

The Parent ego state is typified by behaviours that our parents would have exhibited. The Adult ego state is "autonomously directed towards objective appraisal of reality". The Child ego state is typified by reactions similar to those that we would have made when we were children.

In any of these "states" we are capable of either stimulating a response, or responding to a stimulus. These transactions may be either "crossed", "complementary" or "hidden".

## Complementary transactions

For the purposes of this discussion, two individuals, $X$ and $Y$ will be represented in their ego

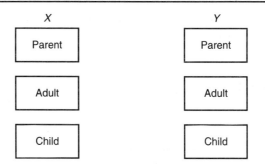

**Figure 1.1.** Ego states.

states (Figure 1.1). For the purposes of this exercise, $X$ is assumed to be the student, whilst $Y$ is the practitioner teacher.

$X$: "The experience on this unit has been badly organised."
$Y$: "I know: I've been saying exactly the same thing for months."

With this exchange, both $X$ and $Y$ are manifesting Parent ego states (Figure 1.2).
 Alternatively (Figure 1.3):

$X$: "I have waited a long time to receive confirmation of my programme, but I appreciate the pressures you are under."
$Y$: "That's very understanding. We are a very busy department."

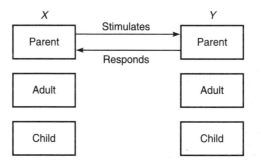

**Figure 1.2.** Complementary transaction (Parent–Parent).

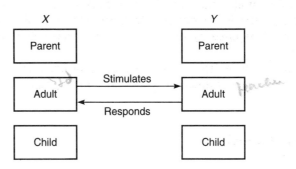

**Figure 1.3.** Complementary transaction (Adult–Adult).

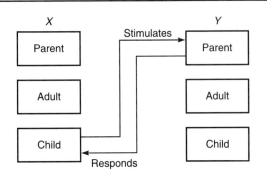

**Figure 1.4.** Complementary transaction (Child–Parent).

Finally (Figure 1.4):

*X*: "No one has taught me anything here and my Finals are in three weeks".
*Y*: "Oh dear, I'm sure we can sort something out for you."

As long as the transactions are complementary (any of the above), the communication will continue. It should always be remembered that often, the "response" can act as a stimulus to the other person to continue the interaction. Not all transactions are this straightforward, and the problem of interacting with someone in an incompatible (to our own) ego state needs to be considered.

## Crossed transactions

When a crossed transaction occurs, the communication between the two parties will either cease, or undergo disturbance in some way. Thus:

*X*: "I haven't had my project marked yet".
*Y*: "So why didn't you remind me before instead of waiting until I'm due to go home".

In this interaction, *X* has made a reasoned statement concerning an unmarked project (Adult). The teacher has responded in a mode other than Adult (Parent) (Figure 1.5). Conflict will therefore occur until a "realignment" to a complementary pattern takes place (if it ever does!)

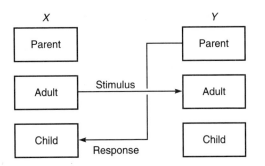

**Figure 1.5.** Crossed transaction (*X–Y*, Adult–Adult; *Y–X*, Parent–Child).

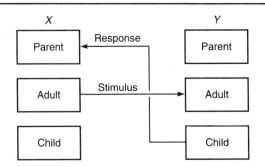

**Figure 1.6.** Crossed transaction ($X$–$Y$, Adult–Adult; $Y$–$X$, Child–Parent).

Alternatively, $Y$ could react to the same question in a child ego state (Figure 1.6), for instance:

"It's not my fault you haven't got it, why can't someone else sort it out for a change?"

Care must be taken to interpret both the message and the "ego state" so that conflict does not occur, by giving a response incompatible with the stimulus. It may happen that the message has a hidden meaning (ulterior transaction). For instance:

"It's probably just me, but I don't see how this can be achieved". (Adult)

could really mean

"That's a ridiculous idea!" (Parent)

Conflict may therefore arise if the reply consists of a Parent-type explanation, with the result that the questioner may feel that he is being "talked down to". A more satisfactory reply could have been to ask the questioner exactly where they see the problem, hence making them reveal their true "ego state".

## Facilitating effective communication skills

In one attempt to teach junior student nurses communication skills, Barnes (1983) reported an incident where hostility expressed by the students took the researchers completely by surprise. It is perhaps, on reflection, not surprising as the author goes on to state that in the early stages of "training", the one area the nurses felt they could safely ignore was that of relating to patients, presumably because they considered this to be a basic human skill.

Effective communication does appear to be a goal which is often not achieved within the realms of patient care (Ley, 1982). Interestingly, those staff who exhibited certain non-verbal behaviours (principally reducing the interpersonal space) were perceived as the most effective teachers.

If the research is to be believed, it would appear that innovative and early attempts to facilitate communication skills need to be made, and that such attempts should offer a broad range of experiences to the learner.

## Using reflection

Reflective practice as described by Boud *et al.* (1985) is a retrospective process concerned with thinking about action, and such a process is in three stages:

1. Reframe the experience through discussion with others (peer group, trained staff and teachers) and purposive thought.
2. Work through the experience using positive feelings and dealing with negative feelings that will prevent effective reflection. In terms of communication, look at the positive aspects of the encounter, or at least what was learned.
3. Re-evaluate the experience and integrate new skills and knowledge.

This form of student centred approach to communication skills should help to overcome some of the difficulties encountered by some authors who have encountered hostility using more traditional approaches.

A word of caution is needed, however, when using such an approach. Firstly, experience should be organised to facilitate the use of reflection as a continuous process. Reflection at the end of an allocation will only have limited uses in this instance.

Secondly, it may be a good idea to make such exercises specific, so that rather than looking at communication skills globally, they could be looked at, for instance after the student has admitted a patient, or following discussions about discharge.

## Using groups

The process of participating in small group work as a way of developing the individual's communication skills has been identified (Glendon and Ulrich, 1992). These skills include disagreeing without stifling new ideas and participating in discussions with others. The peer influence would appear to play a major role in this development, and strategies which combine this sort of activity in the course of undertaking more structured work will usually develop these skills further.

## Teaching style and communication

Using predominantly teacher-centred styles of teaching, such as the formal lecture, will invariably inhibit further development of communication skills. As far as learning communication skills as a subject is concerned, the student's individual learning style should be ascertained, for instance by utilising Kolb's Learning Cycle (Kolb, 1984), and experience planned accordingly. For a full account of this theory the reader is directed to Chapter 5, on learning theories.

One particular style of teaching which has been highlighted as being useful in enhancing communication skills is team teaching. Team teaching can be described as "the active participation of two or more teachers in the planning, preparation, teaching and evaluation of a lesson or a series of lessons" (Minardi and Riley, 1990).

Its uses in the clinical area are not as restricted as the above definition suggests, and it often provides effective support for those involved in the facilitation of the session. Most sessions can be planned and delivered by two or more colleagues on a unit, thus adding different perspectives and even relieving the monotony of single teacher sessions. Teaching methods such as discussion, group work, case studies, games, demonstrations and seminars all lend themselves particularly well to team teaching.

# Summary

During any face-to-face encounter, the type of body language exhibited can make a difference to how a message is interpreted, sometimes regardless of the words that are actually used.

Non-verbal leakage is the process of physical responses which are conveying a different message to the words being used at the time.

The distance between two people has been found to have an effect on the interaction that takes place, and indeed the situation and relationship of the participants will usually determine this distance in the first place (Hall, 1979).

Interference with the communication process is a common phenomenon, and is frequently termed "noise".

Encoding refers to the process of converting an idea into symbols (words). Conversely, decoding is the process by which we translate words back into ideas.

Berne (1964), in discussing the interactions between individuals, described a "system of feelings accompanied by a set of coherent behaviour patterns". These he termed ego states, of which there are three: Parent, Adult and Child.

Reflective practice as described by Boud *et al.* (1985) is a retrospective process concerned with thinking about action.

The process of participating in small group work as a way of developing the individual's communication skills has been identified (Glendon and Ulrich, 1992).

Using predominantly teacher-centred styles of teaching, such as the formal lecture, will invariably inhibit further development of communication skills.

Team teaching can be described as "the active participation of two or more teachers in the planning, preparation, teaching and evaluation of a lesson or a series of lessons" (Minardi and Riley, 1990).

# Suggested activities

## Activity 1

The purpose of this exercise is for you to identify body language that is used to exhibit listening and non-listening behaviours; the exercise is in two parts. To complete it, you should form groups of three and divide the group into one speaker, one listener and and one observer. You will each have the opportunity to play all of these roles as the exercise is repeated.

### Part 1

The speaker and listener should position their chairs as though they were about to have a normal conversation. The observer should be a small distance away but in a position where he/she can comfortably observe all that is going on.

*Speaker*.   You should speak for approximately five minutes about events that took place during the last week of your previous job.

*Listener*.   You should listen to the conversation and respond appropriately.

*Observer*.  You should, without comment, observe the listener during this exercise and note any behaviours that indicate to you that he/she is listening or not listening to the conversation. You should make notes of your observations below.

Change roles and repeat this exercise exactly as above once more.

Come back together as a whole group to discuss your observations and to identify any other non-verbal behaviours which indicate listening.

*Part 2*

Form the same groups as above and adopt the role that you have not yet experienced. You should repeat the exercise as before, except this time, the speaker and listener should take account of the listening behaviours that we have just discussed and consciously try to adopt them.

This can be very useful when you are dealing with staff, patients, relatives or colleagues. In fact, it is useful to know whether someone is being truthful at work or in your personal lives.

It can also be useful if you are feeling very anxious but you wish to appear cool, calm and collected. With practice, it is possible to control your non-verbal behaviour at these times so that you actually appear calm even though you are in an inner-turmoil.

## Activity 2

In this exercise you will be divided into pairs. One person will be the questioner and the other the respondent. At the commencement of the exercise, all respondents will be taken aside and given "secret" instructions, namely who will tell the truth when questioned and who will not. Upon their return, the questioner will be requested to ask the following questions.

1. Why did you decide to enter a career in nursing?
2. Why did you choose this hospital?
3. Which aspects of this job give you pleasure?
4. Which aspects of this job do you dislike?
5. What do you hope to do in the future?

At the end of the exercise, the questioner must quantify a decision as to whether the truth has been told or not! A group discussion should follow.

## Activity 3

As a simple exercise, watch people around you, possibly in a rest room or in a canteen, who are engaged in conversation. If possible, try to choose people whom you know are friends, and watch how similar the posture is for each party.

# References

An asterix indicates a standard text or article.

*Argyle, M. (1983) *The Psychology of Interpersonal Behaviour*, 4th edn. London: Penguin.

Attwell, P. (1974) Ethnomethodology since Garkinkel. *Theory and Society*, **1**, 179–210.

Barnes, D.M. (1983) Teaching communication skills to student nurses – an experience. *Nurse Education Today*, **32**, 45–48.

*Berne, E. (1964) *Games People Play*. New York: Penguin.

Bernstein, B. (1961) Social class and linguistic

development: a theory of social learning. In A.H. Halsey *et al*. (eds), *Education, Economy, and Society*. New York: Free Press.

Boud, D., Keogh, R., and Walker, D. (eds) (1985) *Reflection: Turning Experience into Learning*. London: Kogan Page.

Ekman, P. (1972) Universals and cultural differences in facial expressions of emotion. In: *Nebraska Symposium on Motivation*. University of Nebraska Press. (Quoted in Argyle (1983).)

Ekman, P. (1982) Methods for measuring facial action. In K.R. Scherer and P. Ekman (eds) *Handbook of Methods in Nonverbal Behaviour Research*. Cambridge University Press.

Ekman, P. and Friesen, W.V. (1969) The repertoire of non-verbal behavior: categories, origins, usage and coding. *Semiotics*, 1, 49–98.

*Elkin, F. (1945) The soldier's language. *American Journal of Sociology*, **51**, 414–422.

Exline, R.V., Parades, A., Gottheil, E. and Winkelmayer, R. (1979) Gaze patterns of normals and schizophrenics retelling happy, sad and angry experiences. In C.E. Izard (ed.) *Emotions in Personality and Psychopathology*. New York: Plenum.

Glendon, K. and Ulrich, D. (1992) Using cooperative learning strategies. *Nurse Educator*, **17**(4), 37–40.

Hall, E.T. (1979) Proxemics. In S. Weitz (ed.) *Non Verbal Communication: Readings with Commentary*, 2nd edn. New York: Oxford University Press.

Hildreth, A.M., Derogatis, L. and McCusker, K. (1971) Body buffer zone and violence: a reassessment and confirmation. *American Journal of Psychiatry*, **127**, 77–81.

Kendon, A. (1967) Some functions of gaze direction in social interaction. *Acta Psychologica*, **26**, 22–63.

Kendon, A. (1982) Organisation of behaviour in face to face interaction. In K.R. Scherer and P. Ekman (eds) *Handbook of Methods in Nonverbal Behaviour Research*. Cambridge University Press.

Kolb, D. (1984) *Experiential Learning: experience as a source of learning and development*. Englewood Cliffs, Prentice Hall.

Lantz, D. and Stefflre, V. (1964) Language and cognition revisited. *Journal of Abnormal and Social Psycholgy*, **69**, 471–481.

Ley, P. (1982) Giving information to patients. In J.R. Eiser (ed) *Social Psychology and Behavioural Medicine*. New York: Wiley.

Minardi, H.A., and Riley, M.J. (1990) The use of team teaching for communication skills training in nurse education. *Nurse Education Today*, **11**, 57–64.

*Morris, D. (1977) *Manwatching – a Field Guide to Human Behaviour*. London: Jonathan Cape.

# Suggested reading

Argyle, M. (1983) *The Psychology of Interpersonal Behaviour*, 4th edn. London: Penguin.
(See Chapter 2 for an account of verbal and non-verbal communication.)

Berne, E. (1964) *Games People Play*. New York: Penguin.
(A very readable text on transactional analysis by its originator.)

Scherer, K.R. and Ekman, P. (eds) (1982) *Handbook of Methods of Non-verbal Behaviour Research*.

(See Chapter 1 for an excellent introduction to investigating non-verbal behaviour.)

Morris, D. (1977) *Manwatching – a Field Guide to Human Behaviour*. London: Jonathan Cape.
(An excellent book which covers the subject of non-verbal communication. See in particular the sections dealing with non-verbal leakage and displacement activities.)

# chapter two

# Attitudes and learning

## Introduction

The term "attitude" crops up frequently in education, but of course it is also a word in common usage. In psychological terms, the importance of attitudes, their formation, and how they may be changed cannot be overemphasised when examining human behaviour.

In education terms, the subject of attitudes requires our attention for three reasons.

1. Firstly, if learning can be described as a more or less permanent change of behaviour and if attitudes direct behaviour, then an immediate link can be seen that requires closer examination.
2. Secondly, and possibly more urgent, we need to clarify exactly what an attitude actually is because of its diverse usage in every-day conversation.
3. Finally, attitudes are frequently assessed, and without a complete understanding of their characteristics this may not be accomplished with any certainty, or indeed fairness.

*Values* are frequently discussed alongside the subject of attitudes with some justification. A value is a belief that something is good and desirable (Haralambos, 1985). The relationship to attitudes is apparent although values cannot be observed directly. Society relies on individuals sharing norms in order that it can cooperate and work together, conversely, individuals within a society with different values will be striving towards vastly different goals. For instance, if we take the case of a group of nurses working in care of the elderly, if the values shared by some are that their clients are an important and integral part of the community then their care will be directed towards this end. If another part of the group believe that the elderly are an encumbrance then their nursing care would differ accordingly.

## What is an attitude?

Several definitions of attitudes exist, although for our purposes, we will use that of Allport (1935), who described an attitude as: "A mental and neural state of readiness, organised through experience, exerting a directive or dynamic influence upon the individual's response to all objects and situations with which it is related".

The picture does, however, appear to be rather more complicated than upon first inspection. Does, for instance an attitude towards an object, person or situation always become obviously manifested in the individual's behaviour? Since we cannot observe an attitude directly, but can only observe behavioural manifestations, can we be certain that we have been able to pinpoint an attitude correctly? In order to consider the possible consequences of these questions, it may be helpful to examine the following case study:

Jo Smith had been employed as a Registered Nurse at the Colshire Hospital for ten years following her training, and in that time she had not undergone any further training and had not done any further study. Her manager, on deciding to revitalise an existing Individualised Patient Care System which was showing few signs of being effective, asked Jo to be part of a group that would undergo a short education programme (two hours a week for seven weeks) and subsequently to help relaunch an improved system.
   In the first two weeks of the education programme, Jo was observed as being rather quiet during the sessions, although she did occasionally take part in the discussions. After the first week, she completed the reading required for the week's session, although she missed the third and fourth sessions. Before the fifth session took place, Jo was raising doubts as to whether such a system should be used in the hospital, and based her argument on stories she had heard (second-hand) from other hospitals.
   Upon hearing an account of Jo's apparent mutiny, and her non-attendance of the education sessions, her manager concluded that Jo had a "poor attitude" towards Individualised Patient Care, and should be replaced on the project team with immediate effect.

The question that we really need to consider is whether the manager was justified in the conclusions that she reached with regard to Jo's attitude. Like many situations in life, one situation is often tied up with others, and this case is no exception. In this instance, at least three events were occurring simultaneously, all of which were related to Individualised Patient Care. These were:

1. Jo was part of a project team which would implement change.
2. Jo was expected to undergo an education programme which included some study.
3. Jo would have to change some of her own practices.

If Allport's definition is to be believed, then Jo would have an attitude to each of these situations, not just to Individualised Patient Care, and that somewhere behavioural manifestations would occur, but because all three events were linked to the project, it might (but not always) prove difficult to ascertain the precise object of the "poor" attitude. In fact, Jo (as it later transpired) had many negative experiences in education, which had left her with a dread of studying. Not wanting to admit what she saw as a weakness, Jo's attitude was shown indirectly by not turning up to further sessions, and by casting doubt on the project, thus leading to her removal from the project team.
   It would seem that to state that we can observe an attitude by the behaviour that is manifested is true, but is fraught with complexities. At this juncture, it is perhaps advisable to "dissect" an attitude and see how it is made up.

# Components of an attitude

An attitude can be viewed as having three components (Secord and Backman, 1964):

1. Cognitive
2. Affective
3. Behavioural

## The cognitive component

The cognitive component is the rational part of an attitude and defines where the attitude is directed towards (object or situation). The cognitive component therefore could be said to consist of our knowledge about an object situation or person although such knowledge will frequently be incomplete. The cognitive component of our attitude has also been described as our beliefs or ideas (McDavid and Harari, 1974).

## The affective component

The affective part of an attitude consists of the feelings that we may have towards the object or situation. We may feel favourably, unfavourably, or perhaps have no particularly strong feelings in either direction and may be very deep-rooted. To put it another way, the emotional or affective component of attitude actually refers to our liking or disliking of the attitude object (Jaspars, 1978).

## The behavioural component

The behavioural (or conative) component of an attitude refers to our tendency we have to behave in a certain way towards the attitude object. Approach tendencies may develop if we have positive feelings towards a particular attitude object, and are manifested by behaviours which will bring us into closer contact with the object or person. The converse is clearly true with negative feelings, in which we will have a tendency to behave in such a way as to distance ourselves from the object (avoidance tendencies). The association between this component of our attitudes and motivation is a strong one as it can be seen that it will direct our behaviour.

This "three component theory" of attitudes brings with it, for many theorists, the assumption that all three components are consistent with each other; in other words, if we have positive beliefs, it will give us positive feelings, which will lead to positive actions. In the first instance, this is probably extremely difficult to observe in real life, as it is difficult to dissect out a specific attitude which is responsible for a specific behaviour, but rather a complex matrix of attitudes is involved in a complex set of behaviours.

There is, however, some evidence to suggest that such a consistency does exist (Campbell, 1963) and as Jaspars (1978) points out the idea that cognitive and affective components of attitude being related leads to attempts to change people's feelings towards certain objects or situations by introducing new information about them.

## The expectancy-value model

The expectancy-value model assumes that expectations are a key feature of attitudes and that the attitude object is viewed as being useful or otherwise to the individual's goals and further to their values. The explanation as to what is meant by cognitive and affective components also differs with this theory, with the cognitive component being defined as a section of associations between the object of attitude and certain attributes or goals (Jaspars, 1978) and the effective component as the evaluation of the associated goals or attributes.

# Attitude formation:

Attitudes are not formed exclusively from one source or another, but rather in a number of ways.

1. The most obvious way is by direct experience, and indeed attitudes based on direct experience are the most accurate.
2. Attitudes are also formed from second-hand knowledge (from other people, television or reading).
3. Attitude formation may also be strongly correlated with our upbringing and the attitudes of our parents, near family and later, peers.

The attitudes that a child has do not, however, solely emerge as a result of copying (modelling) the behaviour and attitudes of others. The whole process of upbringing is a complex system of factors which may and usually does include frequent use of rewards for certain behaviours and lack of reward or punishment for undesirable behaviours. These forms of early conditioning cannot be ignored when discussing attitude formation and it may be worthwhile at this juncture also to mention that indirect experience (in the form of being told by parents that something is good or bad, e.g. do not talk to strangers because it could be very dangerous) has a vital part to play in the early life of any individual.

# Measuring attitudes

The measurement of attitudes has been attempted on an informal basis both in education and in management. The difficulties that can be encountered in trying to ascertain the individual attitude(s) responsible for a certain behaviour have already been discussed above.

It would seem likely therefore, that a more meticulous, analytical approach than just asking, for instance, a generic question such as "what is the nurse's attitude towards parents?", is required.

One such measurement which is in common usage is the Likert Scale (Likert, 1932). It should be pointed out that several things may go astray even by using this method and although a brief account is given on how a Likert Scale is constructed, these cautions should be borne in mind:

1. The statements used in the questionnaire may be poorly constructed.
2. Truthful answers may not be given.
3. Wrong conclusions may be drawn from the results due to lack of experience on the part of the researcher.
4. Underlying attitudes which may explain someone's behaviour may not have been covered on the scale.

Naturally much depends on the experience and expertise of the researcher involved and such a task should not be undertaken lightly.

## Constructing a Likert Scale:

As with any testing procedure the construction of a Likert Scale cannot be done at random. Likert himself first constructed the scale with many items relating to the same issue. These items were then administered to a group of judges who were required to indicate their own attitudes by responding to all the items on a five-point scale. Generally, responses at the two ends of the scale were shown to have more discriminative power than those at the centre (neutral) by implication, therefore these responses are more likely to yield accurate information about someone's attitudes.

**Table 2.1.**  Structure of a Likert Scale

| Statement | Strongly agree | Agree | Neutral | Disagree | Strongly disagree |
|---|---|---|---|---|---|
| The personal tutor is a mentor to the student | | | | | |
| The personal tutor will be available at all times | | | | | |
| The personal tutor will enable student independence | | | | | |

The Likert Scale therefore consists of a number of statements (previously tested as above) relating to an issue and the individual is asked to repond to each statement in one of five ways. These responses will come under the categories of "strongly agree", "agree", "neutral", "disagree" and "strongly disagree". For the purposes of our discussion we will look at a very abridged, hypothetical Likert Scale concerning the attitudes of nurse teachers to the "Personal Tutor Role" (Table 2.1).

The Likert scale, as can be deduced, can be used effectively (if constructed properly) in measuring an individual's attitudes as part of an assessment procedure. Alternatively, it can have a far wider use in determining the attitudes of a group of people towards a certain issue in order to formulate decisions and policies most acceptable to that group.

# Cognitive dissonance (Festinger, 1957)

The notion that attitudes should be consistent towards an object or person, and that this is reflected in our behaviour, is perhaps an ideal. Festinger proposed that there are times when we may have to act in a manner contrary to our beliefs. When this occurs (namely when we no longer have cognitive consistency) then we experience conflict. Of course, most of us do things at times that we do not like or believe in, such as being friendly to an unwelcome guest. This does not normally pose much of a problem as the situation is very short term. If on the other hand, we have to behave inconsistently with our beliefs for a longer period of time then problems will usually occur, e.g. a mentor who already has a full workload being told that they have to take on an extra student.

Cognitive dissonance can therefore be seen as an uncomfortable situation which the individual must resolve one way or the other. This can be done in several ways all of which will be substantially unconscious. For instance:

1. The attidude toward the student could become very negative, leading the mentor to believe that they were not worth spending time on.
2. We may form affiliations with others who feel similarly aggrieved.
3. We may start to invent reasons as to why certain tasks should not be completed.
4. We may enter into a conflict situation with the person who originally asked us to take on the extra work.

In terms of trying to bring some equilibrium into the work situation (Adams, 1963), we may:

1.  Reduce the amount of effort that we put into a job.
2.  Attempt to gain more benefits from the job.
3.  Distort the situation mentally by, for instance, minimising the importance of the workload.
4.  In extreme circumstances, we may even leave the job.

Most of all the characteristic that typifies the outcome of cognitive dissonance is attitude change and one of the most powerful instruments involved in such change is communication.

# Communication and attitude change

The characteristics of both the "sender" and "recipient", in relation to attitude change, will be discussed here, as will the mode of transmission and the structure of the message. If we wish to draw the distinction between the relatively straightfoward transmission of a message, and a communication capable of changing an attitude, then we need to view such communication in terms of its ability to persuade an individual student or group.

## The sender

The individual who is communicating the message has an influence over the effectiveness of the message, and one of the reasons for not listening is that the "sender" of the message is not liked, for one reason or other. If we assume that one of the major functions of education is to change attitudes then it can be seen that the relationship between the student and the mentor/preceptor is of vital importance.

It perhaps comes as no suprise that we are more likely to take notice of the message if we perceive the communicator as being attractive, either physically, or in relation to personality. Admiration for, and even identification or similarity with the "sender" may actually prove to be more persuasive than the message content itself (Newcomb, 1961). The personality of the sender will naturally have an effect on changing attitudes, but in this case it seems logical to suppose that it is the perceived personality of the sender that will give credibility to the message rather than the sender's actual personality.

Naturally, credibility does not depend only upon whether we perceive the sender as being confident or pleasant (or indeed attractive), but they must also be perceived as being credible in terms of their knowledge and expertise, although this effect is diminished when the recipient is strongly involved with the attitude object being discussed (Johnson and Scileppi, 1969). For instance, many teachers of nursing may find it easier to change the attitudes of ward staff in a subject that the ward staff feel they have little knowledge of (such as a different speciality), than to change an attitude towards something that they do everyday and consider themselves expert in.

## The message

Obviously, the sender of the message can have little effect on changing attitudes if the message they are giving is of little worth. It is therefore reasonable to say that the content of the message is of vital importance, but also it cannot be ignored that the message must be attended to, and subsequently understood. The factors that may prevent this have already been discussed in part (this chapter), and this will be looked at further when discussing the "recipient". Amongst other factors, the encoding and decoding of the message is of major importance.

The evidence to support or refute various aspects of the importance of message structure and content is considerable, and at times contradictory (Jaspars, 1978). Some facts, however, do appear to emerge as being significant to attitude change.

## One- and two-sided arguments

To state that the message should be directed towards the cognitive or affective components does not tell us how this may be achieved, and therefore some consideration of this aspect is necessary. The presentation of facts, with or without an emotional slant will need to be structured in such a way as to take account of the existing attitudes of the "recipient". If, for instance, the "recipient" is well disposed towards the "sender", a one-sided argument may be more effective than a two-sided argument which may prove to be more productive when directed towards a more indifferent or antagonistic audience, and the opposing argument needs to be faced and attacked (Niven, 1989). The two-sided argument is also of use when talking to individuals who are familiar with the subject matter.

## Drawing conclusions from the argument

The question then arises as to what conclusions the audience or individual may come to, following the presentation of the argument. Put another way, should the recipients be given the conclusion, or should they be left to form their own? In looking at this problem, we have to consider that we are all individuals with unique perceptions and experiences, and that a conclusion obvious to one person may not be obvious to another. It therefore seems likely that the message should carry its own conclusions in order to be effective in changing attitudes (Haskins, 1966).

## The recipient

Many of the factors which have already been discussed will depend upon the perceptions and experiences of the recipient of the message, and therefore it can be seen immediately that the recipient is a key factor. Taking this individual approach to interpersonal communication should prevent us from making unwarranted generalisations, so that instead of, for instance repeating the same information with regard to orientation programmes, they should be tailored to the individual. Put another way, do we teach a subject to junior colleagues without adapting it to meet their individual needs?

The chances are that most of us will have preconceived ideas as to how a subject may be broached from a subject matter viewpoint, but have paid little attention to the factors which may affect the recipient's use and interpretation of it. This is not intended as a damning criticism, as it is frequently impossible to know sufficient details about our audience in advance in order to plan effectively; this may only be achieved when we meet the individual.

The fact remains, as we may have observed from our everyday lives, that some people are more susceptible to persuasion than others. McGuire (1969) suggested that self-esteem may be related to the amount of attitude change that takes place, inasmuch as a high self-esteem may be positively related to understanding the message, but negatively related to undergoing attitude change as a result.

# Prejudice

If we make the fairly safe assumption that we form generalisations about specific objects, groups or even individuals based on very little concrete knowledge and experience, then it is not beyond reason that these generalisations may be faulty and inflexible. Bad experiences in certain situations may lead us to form such inflexible generalisations and may even lead us to apply these to a wider group of objects or individuals.

For instance, if we act as a mentor to a student for the first time, and that student (and subsequently two or three others), causes us anguish and embarrassment, then we may begin to predict (quite unreasonably) that all students will be the same. This could be applied to virtually any situation in life and, it has to be said, is virtually impossible to avoid.

*Prejudice* is therefore a specific type of attitude described by Allport (1954) as "an antipathy based on a faulty and inflexible generalisation directed towards a group as a whole or towards an individual because he is a member of that group". It must be reiterated that our attitudes will direct our behaviour and it could be said that we make predictions as to the outcomes of certain situations based on the generalisations that we have made from the past. If we now take the argument one step further, it can be seen that such predictions and the associated behaviours that we may exhibit may be unwarranted. Naturally in the absence of inflexibility (or in this case in the absence of prejudice) the consequences are not usually dire.

The major factor that distinguishes a prejudice from more "normal" attitudes is its apparent lack of permeability to new information which may serve to disprove the generalisations that have been made. For example, we may be prejudiced against nurses that have certain characteristics such as those undertaking different forms of education than we did. We may ascribe the characteristic "disinterested" to the first two or three that we meet, and we could well be correct in our judgements. If the experience of working with such individuals is unpleasant, we may (but by no means certainly) form an inflexible approach to future individuals, regardless of whether they are "disinterested" or not, and we will behave accordingly towards them.

One of the distinguishing factors of a prejudice is that if the evidence disproves our generalisation, we will find another reason for it, or be of the opinion that they are the exception to the rule, or just ignore the evidence altogether. On the other hand, a prejudice will direct us to seek evidence, no matter how flimsy, that our assumptions were correct in the first place. This stereotyping is characteristic of a prejudice and may be either in a positive or negative direction.

It is naturally assumed by many that a prejudice is directed against an object or individual, although Reich and Adcock (1976) point out that prejudice can be considered as a continuum from extremely favourable to extremely unfavourable.

## Effects of prejudice

Taking into account the fact that a prejudice may work in either direction, Philp (1983) identified basic sources of error which he terms as "halos or horns". The halo effect in terms of attitudes has the effect of overrating the individual's performance and may stem from either observing their past performance or from observing similar individuals' performance. The horn effect, conversely, emerges when the individual's record of performance is underrated. Philp goes on to point out that this may emerge from the non-conformity of the individual involved, or when the assessor is particularly perfectionist in nature. Of course, if the individual and the mentor/preceptor are highly compatible in terms of interest, background and possibly even personality, then it is more likely that the "halo effect" will emerge.

None of us likes to admit that we are unreasonable in our judgements of others, even less that we may be prejudiced towards certain individuals or groups. We may indeed be able to offer convincing justifications for what other people may see as unreasonable assumptions. We should be aware though that we all have prejudices to some degree and that these may affect the way we treat students. It is not unreasonable for an individual to recognise this facet and to ask another individual to take over their role of mentor/preceptor if they feel that their own judgements may be biased. The only barrier to this entirely reasonable action is the reluctance for one person to admit their feelings to another. This may be due to a working environment that is not conducive to self-disclosure.

# Summary

A value is a belief that something is good and desirable (Haralambos, 1985).

Allport (1935), described an attitude as: "A mental and neural state of readiness, organised through experience, exerting a directive or dynamic influence upon the individual's response to all objects and situations with which it is related."

An attitude can be viewed as having three components (Secord and Backman, 1964):

1. Cognitive.
2. Affective.
3. Behavioural.

The cognitive component is the rational part of an attitude and defines where the attitude is directed towards (object or situation). The affective part of an attitude consists of the feelings that we may have towards the object or situation. The behavioural (or conative) component of an attitude refers to the tendency we have to behave in a certain way towards the attitude object.

The expectancy-value model assumes that expectations are a key feature of attitudes and that attitude object is viewed as being useful or otherwise to the individual's goals and further to their values.

One measurement which is used to measure attitudes is the Likert Scale (Likert, 1932).

Festinger (1957) proposed that there are times when we may have to act in a manner contrary to our beliefs. When this occurs (namely when we no longer have cognitive consistency) then we experience conflict (cognitive dissonance).

If we wish to draw the distinction between the relatively straightfoward transmission of a message, and a communication capable of changing an attitude, then we need to view such communication in terms of its ability to persuade an individual student or group.

Prejudice is a specific type of attitude described by Allport (1954) as "an antipathy based on a faulty and inflexible generalisation directed towards a group as a whole or towards an individual because he is a member of that group".

Philp (1983) identified basic sources of error which he terms as "halos or horns"

# Related Activities

## Activity 1

Construct a Likert Scale, following the example given in Table 2.1. Identify a series of at least 15 positive statements which describe the role of the mentor. Try to include some contentious statements (but not necessarily disagreeable ones), e.g. "The mentor should always be on duty with the student".

Perhaps you could use the results from Activity 1.

## Activity 2

1. Administer the Likert Scale you have constructed to a group of five students working in your speciality (pilot study).
2. Eliminate those items where the majority of responses have been "Neutral" and reconstruct your test with the remaining items.
3. Administer the amended test to a different group of students (obviously there may be a delay between running your pilot and carrying out the final amended test if you need to wait for a new group of students).
4. Examine the results and discuss with your colleagues how the findings can be implemented.

# References

An asterix indicates a standard text or article.

Adams (1963) Towards an understanding of inequity. *Journal of Abnormal and Social Psychology*, **67**, 422–436.

Allport, G.W. (1935) Attitudes. In Murchinson, C.M. (ed.) *Handbook of Social Psychology*. Mass.: Clark University Press.

Allport, G.W. (1954) *The Nature of Prejudice*. Wokingham: Addison-Wesley.

Campbell, D.T. (1963) Social attitudes and other acquired behavioural dispositions. In S. Koch (ed) *Psychology: a Study of a Science*, **vol. 6**. New York: McGraw Hill.

*Festinger, L. (1957) *A Theory of Cognitive Dissonance*. New York: Harper and Row.

Haralambos, M. (1985) *Sociology Themes and Perspectives*, 2nd edn. London: Unwin Heinman.

Haskins (1966) Factual recall as a measure of advertising effectiveness. *Journal of Advertising Research*, **6**, 2–8.

Jaspars, J.M.F. (1978) *Determates of Attitude and Attitude Change*. In, H. Tajfel & C. Fraser (eds.) *Introducing Social Psychology*. Hamondsworth: Penguin.

Johnson and Scilepi (1969) Effects of Ego involvement Conditions of Attitude Change to High and Low Ability Communications. *Journal of Personality and Social Psychology*, **13**, 31–36.

Likert, R. (1932) A Technique for the measurement of attitudes. *Archives of Psychology*, **22**, 1–55.

McGuire, W.J. (1969) The nature of attitudes and attitude change. In G. Lindzey & E. Aronson (eds.) *Handbook of Social Psychology 2nd edn. Vol. 13*. New York, Addison-Wesley.

Newcomb, T.M. (1961) *The Acquaintance Process*. New York: Holt, Rinehart and Winston.

Niven, N. (1989) *Health Psychology – an Introduction for Nurses and other Health Professionals*. London: Churchill Livingstone.

Philp, T. (1983) *Making Performance Appraisal Work*. Maidenhead: McGraw-Hill.

Reich, B. and Adcock, C. (1976) *Values, Attitudes and Behaviour Change*. London: Methuen.

*Secord, P.F. and Backman, C.W. (1964) *Social Psychology*. McGraw-Hill.

# chapter three

# Groups

## Introduction

The study of groups is important to a discussion for a variety of reasons. Firstly, learners are usually members of a large group or cohort, which in turn is usually divided into smaller groups either by the choice of individuals or for education or management reasons. Secondly, the environment in which the learner is gaining experience is usually outside their own system of groups.

In addition to these groups we can all describe many other groups either with an organisational or social function which may have an effect on a learner and the environment in which they operate.

Groups can and do exert considerable influences over most individuals under certain circumstances and therefore it makes sense to consider some aspects of the psychology of groups. In doing so, perhaps some insight may be gained into the behaviour of both the learner and those facilitating their learning. In order to do this the discussion will examine group functions, dynamics, communication, and types of groups with particular reference to those groups which are important in education. Leadership styles are of course inextricably linked to group dynamics and this too will be discussed. Perhaps the most appropriate way to start is to examine briefly the scope of the subject in hand by looking at some of the different types of group.

## Types of groups

Most of us could, without giving too much thought to it, identify two distinct types of group, namely, those which fulfil or (attempt to fulfil) a particular task and those which fulfil a social function. The former type of group is frequently termed a "formal" group and the second type, not surprisingly is known as the "social" group. The classification is by no means as simple as it would first appear and it may be more relevant to describe groups as having either a formal function, or a social function, or indeed both. Naturally, some groups are less permanent than others and once their task has been completed then they will disband, for example project teams, working parties and even interviewing panels.

The groups that have a more permanent basis, such as the ward teams, are more likely to have a social function as well as a formal one by virtue of the time its members spend together on their everyday interactions in the course of their work.

Chell (1989) describes some key characteristics as formal functions:

1. The ability to work on interdependent tasks.
2. The means of generating new ideas and creating new solutions to complex problems.
3. For purposes of liaison and coordination.

4. To facilitate the implementation of complex decisions.
5. As a vehicle for change.
6. To enable the socialisation and training of new members.

Certainly, the organisational groups that we use in our work practice will essentially fulfil all of the above functions. It is relatively easy to take the case of any group, for instance a curriculum planning team, and to see how it fulfils these functions.

When considering education groups the picture is not really that different, although the formal functions are likely to have less of a direct effect on the organisation. In terms of, for instance "buzz" groups, which are used on a very short-term basis, we can see that the functions may be far more specific in terms of generating new ideas in creating solutions and far less specifically a vehicle for change, with the changes in this instance being far less predictable in terms of an end product because the changes may be the effects of learning, rather than, for instance a new curriculum or the effective functioning of a team.

It should be reiterated that the type of functions that a group will fulfil will be largely dependent on the time the groups spend together and the amount of interdependence that occurs, and as such, groups in education tend to have a rather longer life span than those formed during a practice allocation, and have more of a social function.

Chell goes on to describe some social functions, which are relevant to our discussion:

1. They fulfil affiliation needs of friendship, love and support.
2. They define the individual's sense of identity and maintain self-esteem.
3. They enable individuals to establish and test reality through discussion, questioning, talking about events and coming to share perspectives about how those events should be defined.
4. They reduce feelings of insecurity and anxiety, and a sense of powerlessness by reducing uncertainty and providing each member with social support.
5. They enable members to solve problems and accomplish tasks through the group.
6. They are a means of entertainment, alleviating boredom/fatigue, boosting morale and personal satisfaction.
7. They produce the means by which members encounter managerial power.

Many of us can identify our own student groups in the past as having a strong social function, and the support they gave us during new and sometimes daunting learning experiences. To cut the student off completely from their peers can be detrimental to the learning process, and this should be borne in mind when planning a learning experience, particularly where shifts are involved.

# Group atmosphere

Another angle which can be explored in terms of social functions is the *group climate* or atmosphere. This is a very global way of characterising the structural properties of the group and describes some of the attributes of the group; for instance, group climate may be

1. Emotional
2. Social
3. Affiliative
4. Friendly
5. Aggressive
6. Apathetic

The list could actually be much longer, but the underlying climate is the important determining factor when considering what the group can achieve and how they can go about it. It may be that the group with the social bias may be especially effective in giving support to its members during a crisis. A friendly group will probably have a different relationship to teaching staff than will an aggressive group.

Group climate can said to be the general tone of all relationships within the group, and although it is apparently easy to identify on some occasions, it may be virtually impossible to do so on others. However, it is perhaps worth mentioning at this stage that on many occasions where a group could be labelled difficult or aggressive, extreme caution should be exercised, as the group may have been responding to particular novel stimuli or even to particular individuals with whom it came into contact, and that overall no such group climate actually exists.

# Leadership

One important aspect of groups is the concept of leadership. Lewin *et al.* (1939), in a now classic study of boys' clubs, looked at how the leadership approach of their adult leaders varied. The researchers identified three leadership styles:

1. Autocratic
2. Democratic
3. *Laissez-faire*

## The autocratic leader

This leader will tend to make all decisions whether they are needed or not and will usually see that they are adhered to strictly. It should be borne in mind, as with other leadership styles, that this does not necessarily refer to a particular type of personality. In doing this experiment it was found that as far as productivity was concerned the output was good for as long as the leader was present, but the output from the group dropped dramatically in the absence of such a leader.

## The democratic leader

With this style, the leader is aware of taking decisions only after democratic consultation with the group. When the leader was present, the output was not quite as good as with the autocratic leader; however, the output continued to be consistent even in the absence of the leader.

## The *laissez-faire* leader

This leader did not make any decisions unless asked to do so, and when decisions were made they were usually ineffective and lacked direction. The results of this type of leadership were interesting in that, as far as completing a task was concerned, there was a consistently low, poor quality output from the group with, or without the leader. However, this style of leadership was found to be effective when a creative outcome was required.

# Leadership and the learning climate

This description of leadership styles is still commonly used today, although it would be wrong to assume that each of us could fit into any one of these categories. Certainly, as far as this classification is concerned, it would seem reasonable to assume that most of us would fall somewhere between these categories, and would adopt different strategies according to the situation confronting us. Our leadership style could be affected by our personality, our needs, managerial circumstances, the characteristics of the group involved, communication patterns, group size and whether there was any stress or crisis in the situation.

As far as the educational climate is concerned it would seem unlikely that an effective learning environment could be created where an efficient two-way communication pattern could not be maintained, and hence an autocratic style of leadership on the part of whoever is responsible for facilitating learning, could have detrimental effects.

That the leadership style should be approachable and learner orientated (Ogier, 1980) probably comes as no surprise, although the style should also be sufficiently directive for the nature of the work involved. This could lead us to conclude that the democratic style of leadership, at least for the majority of situations, would be most effective, with the *laissez-faire* style lacking direction, and the autocratic style preventing effective two-way communication.

# Leaders and managers

One of the interesting features about the work of Lewin *et al.* is that all the leaders had been appointed by those other than the members of the groups that they ultimately led. This of course is normally the case in any work situation where a manager is appointed to a particular group or area. The argument that presents itself in this context is concerned with the differences between managers and leaders, and this of course will depend very much on the definitions that we give to each one.

If we define a leader as an individual who influences or directs the behaviour of a group of people, it can be seen that this can only be partly fulfilled by an appointed manager whose primary function may be administrative. With regard to the health care team it may be the case that the group itself identifies the manager as its leader, although it may have informally "elected" its own leader who will have considerable influence over the attitudes and behaviour of the group as a whole.

## *Task and social specialists*

It has been suggested that leaders can be classified as task specialists or social specialists (Bales, 1950). A task specialist's aim is primarily to ensure that the job gets done, whereas the social specialist is effective with the group's interpersonal relationships and other social dimensions. This classification could at least go some way to settling the debate on the nature of a manager and a leader, with both being leaders, with the manager being a task-orientated leader and the "leader" being socially orientated. Certainly there is room to argue that each may be an effective leader, and that the distinction is one of definition and the situation in which the leader is attempting to function.

## Contingency theory

One leadership theory that has gained considerable prominence in recent years is the "contingency" theory of leadership proposed by Fiedler (1967). Fiedler suggested that:

> The group's performance will be contingent upon the appropriate matching of leadership style and the degree of favourableness of the group situation for the leader, that is the degree to which the situation provides the leader with influence over the group members.

The model therefore suggests that group performance can be improved either by modifying the leadership style or by modifying the group-task situation. The importance of the relationships within the group and between group members and the leader, the structure of the task in hand, and whether the leader is legitimate in the position that they occupy are all important to Fiedler's contingency theory.

Fiedler attempted to measure the leadership style of an individual indirectly by the use of various scales, the most famous of which is the "Least Preferred Co-worker Scale" (LPC). With this scale respondents are asked to rate the individual with whom they have liked working with the least (past or present) on an evaluative scale (Figure 3.1). On analysis the scales were said to reveal that those achieving a high score have the following characteristics:

1. Concerned with establishing good interpersonal relationships.
2. More considerate than those with a low LPC score.
3. Produce lower levels of anxiety in the group.
4. Tend to separate the person from the job.
5. Establish prominence and self-esteem through good relationships.
6. Task success (or failure) does not usually change their style of leadership significantly.
7. Will further affiliate with the group if satisfaction of need is threatened.

Those individuals with a low LPC score were found to be:

1. Task orientated.
2. Produced high levels of anxiety in the groups they led.
3. Goal orientated.
4. Gained satisfaction through task performance.
5. Could tolerate poor interpersonal relationships.

In summary, it appears that those with a high LPC score were friendly, permissive and accepting, and those with a low LPC score were aloof and task orientated.

Some researchers have pointed towards difficulties in statistical analysis and quantifying their results (Fiedler, 1972) and research is continuing in this area, although it is interesting to note that Lewin *et al.*'s original classification is still used extensively although usually in a more modified form, when describing leadership styles.

## Discussion: who leads?

The effect of leadership styles in the learning environment is a rather complicated one and leads us to surmise who is eligible to be a leader within the student group. We have already briefly considered the role of leadership styles on the part of the ward manager and its possible consequences for the learning environment.

If we consider that the manager is attempting (at least most of the time) to achieve the same goals as their subordinates, then their role as leader could be viewed as legitimate. It can be seen that the leader in this instance is, at least in part, task orientated, in as much as they are attempting to provide high quality patient/client care, and this is in common with the rest of the team. It seems possible, however, that the social function of this particular type of leader may be confined to those staff who are permanent to that work situation and may conceivably exclude the student population who are only there for a short period of time and may be supernumerary.

It is vital therefore that the student group should be able to fulfil this function independently,

| | | |
|---|---|---|
| Pleasant | :—:—:—:— \| —:—:—:— | Unpleasant |
| | 8 7 6 5 \| 4 3 2 1 | |
| Friendly | :—:—:—:— \| —:—:—:— | Unfriendly |
| | 8 7 6 5 \| 4 3 2 1 | |
| Rejecting | :—:—:—:— \| —:—:—:— | Accepting |
| | 1 2 3 4 \| 5 6 7 8 | |
| Helpful | :—:—:—:— \| —:—:—:— | Frustrating |
| | 8 7 6 5 \| 4 3 2 1 | |
| Unenthusiastic | :—:—:—:— \| —:—:—:— | Enthusiastic |
| | 1 2 3 4 \| 5 6 7 8 | |
| Tense | :—:—:—:— \| —:—:—:— | Relaxed |
| | 1 2 3 4 \| 5 6 7 8 | |
| Distant | :—:—:—:— \| —:—:—:— | Close |
| | 1 2 3 4 \| 5 6 7 8 | |
| Cold | :—:—:—:— \| —:—:—:— | Warm |
| | 1 2 3 4 \| 5 6 7 8 | |
| Cooperative | :—:—:—:— \| —:—:—:— | Uncooperative |
| | 8 7 6 5 \| 4 3 2 1 | |
| Supportive | :—:—:—:— \| —:—:—:— | Hostile |
| | 8 7 6 5 \| 4 3 2 1 | |
| Boring | :—:—:—:— \| —:—:—:— | Interesting |
| | 1 2 3 4 \| 5 6 7 8 | |
| Quarrelsome | :—:—:—:— \| —:—:—:— | Harmonious |
| | 1 2 3 4 \| 5 6 7 8 | |
| Self-assured | :—:—:—:— \| —:—:—:— | Hesitant |
| | 8 7 6 5 \| 4 3 2 1 | |
| Efficient | :—:—:—:— \| —:—:—:— | Inefficient |
| | 8 7 6 5 \| 4 3 2 1 | |
| Gloomy | :—:—:—:— \| —:—:—:— | Cheerful |
| | 1 2 3 4 \| 5 6 7 8 | |
| Open | :—:—:—:— \| —:—:—:— | Guarded |
| | 8 7 6 5 \| 4 3 2 1 | |

**Figure 3.1.** Least Preferred Co-worker Scale (Fiedler, 1967).

and if we are to believe the research, then emergent leaders will soon become apparent, although it should be remembered that such a phenomenon may never occur.

The subject of leadership is therefore a contentious one in which several different aspects can be explored. It does, however, present us with another dimension of the structure of groups, and this will be further explored below in the section examining sociometric analysis.

## Group norms and conformity

Groups will invariably have developed their own sets of standards that the members find acceptable and advantageous to maintain. The behaviours that the group demands of its members will naturally depend upon not only the function of the group, but also the group climate and types of members, as well as an almost infinite number of other stable and variable factors.

Possibly one of the most challenging management problems as far as groups are concerned is that norms cannot be imposed on a group from the outside, they have to come from within the group itself. This is particularly important when discussing changes to things which the group has adopted as its norms.

# Sociometry

*Sociometry* is a technique for identifying the structure of groups in terms of the nature of relationships between its members, and was developed by Moreno (1934). To be more specific, sociometry is concerned with the social structure, organisation and positions of individuals within groups, and will indicate the individual's likes/dislikes within the group setting.

The sociometric procedure is designed to produce an objective picture of the relationships within the group and to indicate likes, dislikes, attractions, repulsions, etc., between individuals at a given time. The results of such a procedure must always be confidential and hence should not normally be made available to members of the group.

The procedure itself comprises the investigator asking the individuals within a group a specific question, such as: "who do you like to work with?", along with its opposite: "who do you dislike working with?". The context of the question in terms of the occasion and/or activity involved must always be carefully specified; an individual may choose a different set of people socially to those at work.

## Sociograms

Sociometric data may be recorded on a *sociogram*, which is a diagrammatic representation of the interrelationships within a group. Certain rules can be followed in order to make the sociogram easier to interpret:

1. Individuals are represented by letters or numbers.
2. A circle may represent a female: Ⓐ
3. A triangle may represent a male: △.
4. A continuous line between symbols may indicate attraction.

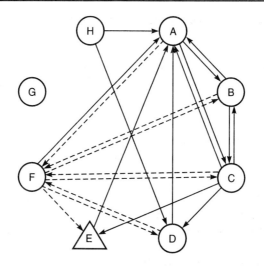

**Figure 3.2.** A sociogram.

5. A broken line between symbols may indicate rejection.
6. An arrow head shows the direction of feeling, e.g.:

A ----------------→ B (A rejects B).
A ————————→ B (A chooses B).

It may now be advantageous to look at the fictitious results of our earlier questions: "Who do you like to work with?" and "Who do you dislike working with?", and to see how this may be represented on the sociogram.

A likes to work with B and C, and dislikes working with F.
B likes to work with A and C, and dislikes working with F.
C likes to work with A, B, D and E, and dislikes working with F.
D likes to work with A, and dislikes working with F.
E likes to work with A.
F likes to work with A, and dislikes working with B, C, D and E.
G makes no choices.
H likes to work with A and D.

Translated into a sociogram, we get the sort of configuration shown in Figure 3.2. Some structures are found time and time again in sociograms, and indeed, are to be seen in our fictitious example. These have been given specific names:

1. Mutual pair – where two individuals choose each other:

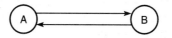

2. Chain structure – where there is a sucession of individuals making non reciprocated choices:

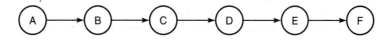

3. Triangle – where three individuals make mutual choices, and this suggests a clique within the group:

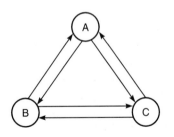

4. Star – this is an individual who many individuals are attracted to, although the "star" may not necessarily reciprocate:

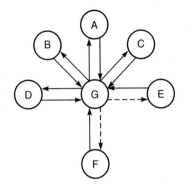

5. Isolate – this individual does not make choices and is not chosen (or rejected).
6. Neglectee – this individual is not chosen by anyone, although they make choices:

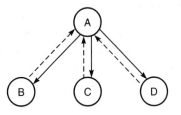

7. Rejectee – this individual is rejected by others and is not chosen by any:

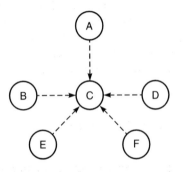

Within the fictitious sociogram in Figure 3.2, try to identify the seven structures described.

## Advantages and disadvantages of the sociogram

It can be seen by looking at the above example that it is fairly easy to read a sociogram without any previous experience, and it is a good way of collecting information and representing it so that many relationships can be seen simultaneously.

Naturally, the observer will wish to know about cliques, people who are being rejected, possible leaders (stars), and generally the popularity of certain individuals, and the degree to which some individuals are rejected or ignored. This in turn will give the observer an idea about group cohesiveness, as well as being able to identify possible areas of conflict.

The concept of cohesiveness is rather difficult to quantify, although a sociometric definition (Lott and Lott, 1965) defines cohesiveness as "that property which is inferred from the number and strength of mutual positive attitudes among the members of the group", and as such may be apparent upon inspection of the data recorded on the sociogram.

A sociogram does, however, have its drawbacks, not least of all the difficulty in interpreting the data if a large number of individuals are involved. A possibly less apparent but crucial disadvantage is that the investigator may be asking inappropriate or insufficient questions in order to gain an overall picture, and indeed, several sociograms may need to be completed for the same group in order to gain an overall impression of the relationships within the group.

Sociometric data do not give reasons for the individuals' choices, and hence if potential conflict areas are found, then further investigations may be required in order to uncover their causes.

## The sociogram in education

The sociogram is, nevertheless, a valuable tool in helping us to gain an insight into the dynamics of the group, and has been used extensively in teaching situations. It can be utilised when making choices in terms of allocations to practice areas, project groups, and indeed any sphere of activity where relationships play an important role.

In terms of those facilitating learners, particularly where the learner is being assessed, it is particularly useful to consider how some individuals may affect others' opinions of the learner (either positively or negatively). For instance: do the cliques tend to reach the same conclusions? Does the group reject or ignore the opinions of a rejectee, neglectee or isolate? Is there objectivity when the "star" behaves in a certain way, or do we gloss over faults and opinions that we may not tolerate in others?

At the end of the chapter, you will be invited to construct a sociogram of your own area, and it may be useful, on your own, to reflect on past incidents and situations in the light of the information gained on the sociogram. Remember, if you ask your group for information, then it must be kept confidential, and if you believe that they may react adversely to being asked, then you should reconsider your decision to investigate the group in this way.

## Communication patterns in the group

Probably one of the most obvious facets of a structural organisation within a group are stable lines of communication. This is not to say that each member of the group interacts equally with everyone else in the group, rather that there is a consistent utilisation of established lines of communication. These lines may be predetermined as in a management or military structure. These structures are commonly termed *communication nets*.

The investigation of these communication nets is complex, particularly when looking at informal or large groups, and hence most experimentation is laboratory based, and will restrict the modes of communication to, for instance, telephone calls or notes. In such experiments, subjects are assigned a task to complete within certain predetermined nets, the main types of which are shown below. It will be noticed that the nets are broadly organised into circles, chains, "Y"s and wheels, and these are illustrated in Figure 3.3.

The circle net involves large numbers of messages being sent, and although being rather slow and cumbersome, lacking leadership, direction and organisation, leads to greater activity and enjoyment by group members. Similar characteristics (although not as extreme) can be attributed to the "chain" configuration. The chain can be described as a broken circle, and participants are said to occupy "peripheral" positions. The wheel configuration, by contrast, concentrates the available channels of communication around one central hub, with the other members of the group being in peripheral positions. The "Y" pattern resembles an adapted wheel and hence shares many of its characteristics, although not to the same extent.

It can therefore be seen that if we just consider the above four nets, then the extreme positions

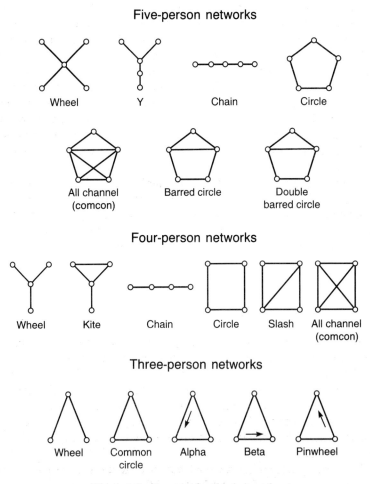

**Figure 3.3.** Communication networks.

in terms of characteristics will be held by the "circle" at one end, and the "wheel" at the other, with the "chain" and "Y" being modified circles and wheels respectively. It should also be mentioned that the more central the position occupied by participants, the more satisfaction is experienced. As for those individuals occupying peripheral positions, they tend to feel uninvolved and not suprisingly derive little satisfaction from their involvement in the group.

If we look at the two extremes in terms of their ability to solve problems effectively, then it has been observed (e.g. Leavitt, 1951), that it is in fact the "wheel" configuration which perpetuates errors, and the "circle" pattern which allows for internal correction of errors.

It will be noticed that one further net has been illustrated, namely the "all channels open" or "comcon" as it is sometimes called. This net allows each member of the group to communicate with every other member directly, and this would appear to be the ideal situation to be in. In reality though, this does not happen, as not all of the available communication channels are used equally, and hence a much simpler structure usually emerges.

# Conclusions

The study of groups has implications for just about every aspect of our social behaviour. The learning environment is no exception. The multitude of interactions that the learner will have in a three-year education programme will mean that they will come into contact with numerous groups, each with their own sets of characteristics and group norms.

In addition to the groups that they temporarily interact with are the more "stable" groups that they are a more permanent part of, and these groups must never be ignored in the planning process. The group climate that the student may find themselves involved in, either on a temporary or permanent basis may affect the amount and quality of learning that may take place. More especially, it has been found that the type of leader has a bearing on the learning environment, and areas that provide experience for students should perhaps consider whether they can utilise Fiedler's concept of either modifying the leadership style or modifying the group-task situation.

The roles of groups in terms of communication skills and as a vehicle for teaching (i.e. group work, etc.) have been discussed elsewhere in the text, and these topics should be read with the information given in this chapter on group climate, etc. Certainly when contemplating the student-centred methods of teaching in which group work is utilised, to ignore the psychology and mechanics of groups as described in this chapter could lead to less than satisfactory results.

# Summary

Two distinct types of group, namely, those who fulfil (or attempt to fulfil) a particular task and those which fulfil a social function can be identified.

The groups that have a more permanent basis, such as the ward teams, are more likely to have a social function as well as a formal one by virtue of the time its members spend together on their every-day interactions on the course of their work.

To cut the student off from their peers completely can be detrimental to the learning process, and this should be borne in mind when planning a learning experience, particularly where shifts are involved.

The "group climate" is a global way of characterising the structural properties of the group and describes some of the attributes of the group.

Lewin, Lippit and White (1939) identified three leadership styles; Autocratic, Democratic and Laissez-faire. An autocratic style of leadership on the part of whoever is responsible for facilitating learning, could have detrimental effects.

It has been suggested that leaders can be classified as task specialists or social specialists (Bales, 1950).

Contingency theory (Fiedler), suggests that group performance can therefore be improved either by modifying the leadership style or modifying the group-task situation.

The behaviours that the group demands of its members will naturally depend upon not only the function of the group, but also the group climate, types of members as well as an almost infinite number of other stable and variable factors.

Sociometry is concerned with the social structure, organisation and positions of individuals within groups, and will indicate the individual's likes/dislikes within the group setting.

One of the most obvious facets of a structural organisation within a group are stable lines of communication. These lines may be predetermined as in a management or military structure, and are commonly termed "communication nets".

# Related Activities

## Activity 1

Construct a sociogram of your ward/unit team. This particular team must have responsibility for learners. The occasion/situation should be "Who do you like working with?" "Who do you dislike working with?".

Naturally, such a procedure can be rather invasive and may actually disrupt group dynamics. If you feel (possibly after you have discussed it with the group) that this will be the case, then you may use your knowledge of the group to devise the sociogram on your own.

When you have completed this activity, try activity 2 which is based on your findings for this activity.

## Activity 2

Referring to the sociogram you have devised, try to think of how the relationships within the group could affect the learning environment.

## Activity 3

Attempt to identify the communication channels in your team. Does one of the "nets" described in this chapter emerge? Having identified the communication channels, discuss with members of the team how communication channels can be improved in order to:

(a) ensure that team members feel part of the decision-making process;
(b) deal with problems effectively.

# References

Bales, R.F. (1950) A Set of categories for the analysis of small group interaction. *American Sociological Review*, **15**, 257–263.

Chell, E. (1989) *The Psychology of Behaviour in Organisations*. London: MacMillan.

Fiedler, F.E. (1967) *A Theory of Leadership Effectiveness*. New York: McGraw-Hill.

Fiedler, F.E. (1972) Personality, motivational systems and behaviour of high and low LPC persons. *Human Relations*, **25**, 391–412.

Leavitt, H.J. (1951) Some effects of certain communication patterns on group performance. *Journal of Abnormal and Social Psychology*, **46**, 38–50.

Lewin, K., Lippett, R. and White, R.K. (1939) Patterns of aggressive behaviour in experimentally created social climates. *Journal of Social Psychology*, **10**, 271–299.

Lott, A.J. and Lott, B.E. (1965) Group cohesiveness as interpersonal attraction. *Psychological Bulletin*, **64**, 259–309.

Moreno, J.L (1934) *Who Shall Survive? A New Approach to the Problems of Interrelations*. Washington, DC: Nervous and Mental Diseases Publishing Co.

Ogier, M.E. (1980) *The Effect of Ward Sisters Management Style upon Nurse Learners*. PhD Thesis, Birkbeck College, London.

# chapter four

# Mentors and preceptors

## Introduction

The subjects of mentorship and preceptorship have been, and still are, the centre of considerable debate. To some authors (Anforth, 1992) the two roles are incompatible, particularly when the preceptorship role has an assessing component. It remains common practice, however, to incorporate the two roles into one under the umbrella terms Mentor, Key Worker or Preceptor.

In this chapter, the commonly accepted attributes and qualities of both mentors and preceptors will be examined in terms of their application to teaching and assessing in the clinical area and to their consequences in some of the more common learning scenarios, e.g. facilitating learning, the counselling role, advocacy and assessment of learning.

It is perhaps a good starting point to offer some definitions of each term to help the reader appreciate the scope of the subject area.

Throughout this chapter, points for discussion will be raised which the reader will be invited to share with colleagues and in order to gain their views as to the appropriateness of their application to the particular area of practice. In carrying out these exercises, the reader may glean that prescriptive roles may not always be appropriate and that some degree of adaptation will always be necessary.

## The mentor

Many terms in education are abused and misunderstood but perhaps nowhere is this more evident than in the use of the term mentor. There are many writers in the education field who have been at pains to point out the unsatisfactory nature of its usage (Palmer, 1987; Morle, 1990) and so it seems appropriate to examine this term briefly in order to provide a framework for later discussion. In doing this, it should be acknowledged that few authors agree on a common definition.

### Definitions

When discussing the mentor, it should be remembered that it must be done in conjunction with the other part of the relationship commonly known as the "mentoree" (Palmer, 1987). By virtue of the fact that the mentoree, who will normally be a student or junior member of staff, has chosen the mentor, it seems logical that the building of the relationship between the two is of crucial importance. Authors such as Burnard (1990) have expressed concern regarding the prescribing of mentors to students, although a rapport may still develop.

Taking it at its most literal, the term mentor is an ancient name derived from Greek mythology referring to the Mentor who cared for Telemachus. The qualities of mentor were those most resembling a "father figure" and in many ways contemporary concepts of the term mentor have not deviated significantly from this notion.

Levinson *et al.* (1978) described the core components of the mentor not only as an exemplar and counsellor but also as teacher, sponsor, developer of skills, developer of intellect and host.

As far as the English National Board (89)17 is concerned, a mentor is

A person selected by the student to assist, befriend, guide, advise and counsel (but who would not normally be involved in the formal supervision or assessment of that particular student) (ENB, 1989).

Anforth (1992), in reviewing the literature (e.g. Barlow, 1991, Burnard, 1990), is concerned that the role of mentor still requires further definition or as Haggerty (1986) maintains it is still a "definition quagmire".

It seems probable that much of the controversy surrounding the role of the mentor, and indeed its very definition, is due to the fact that mentor is too small a title for such a vast concept and that more than one type of mentor exists in the education of nurses, particularly in the clinical area. Palmer (1987) in looking at approaches to mentoring, has identified true mentoring relationships and pseudo mentoring relationships, which are defined in Table 4.1.

**Table 4.1.** Mentoring relationships

| Relationship | Nature |
|---|---|
| 1. Formal mentoring<br>An artificial relationship created for specific purposes that are essentially work related | Programmes are for<br>(i) Specific purposes, functions and aims<br>(ii) Selected individuals; assigned mentors; forced matching of mentors<br>(iii) Possibility for financial incentives for mentors |
| 2. Informal mentoring<br>A naturally chosen relationship for the purposes and functions as determined by the individuals involved. An enabling relationship in professional, personal and emotional terms | No defined programmes<br>Less specific purposes and functions<br>Self-selection by individuals; shared wish to work together; no explicit gains for mentor |
| 3. Pseudo mentoring<br>Quasi/partial mentoring – created for a specific purpose that is essentially work related<br>Induction/orientation programmes | Mentoring approaches in appearance only as suggested in academic involvement with thesis preparation<br>Specific tasks, organisational issues of short duration |

*Source*: Palmer (1987).

# Mentoring role

The diversity of different programmes to prepare individuals for the mentoring role is in many ways dependent upon the definition of mentor adopted by the institution concerned. Certainly in the past (e.g. Lee, 1991), the role of mentor and assessor were sometimes combined and this naturally would affect the nature of the relationship.

Where the mentoring role, as defined earlier, is utilised (e.g. ENB, 1989), an essentially non-threatening relationship is essential in order that the essence of the mentoring expectations is not damaged. One key area that has been identified in numerous studies into the effectiveness of education in clinical practice is that of stress and therefore some discussion of this topic is required.

# Stress – the learner and the mentor

Perhaps some indication as to the relevance of stress to clinical education can be gleaned from studies into reasons for students leaving training and into possible relationships between stress and low self-esteem. One of the roles of the mentor, by virtue of the relationship which has been built up, is to recognise the effect that stress is having on their mentoree.

## Stress and attrition

The number of nurses leaving training has long been a matter of concern to professional nurses both in education and in practice. Further, the reaction of nursing bodies to this and a multitude of other factors (e.g. UKCC, 1993) has been to revise dramatically the pattern of organisation and delivery of nurse education curricula.

The reasons why students leave training have been investigated on numerous occasions, and the results have yielded some interesting results. Fogg (1989) found that reasons given for leaving fell broadly under the following categories:

1. Trained staff were seen as uncaring, traditional, autocratic and lacking awareness of learners' needs.
2. Academic stimulation was lacking in clinical areas and department of education.
3. Maturity of learners was not recognised.
4. There was a lack of supervision and clinical objectives were not met.
5. There was a lack of support from personal tutors.
6. Learners developed a negative self-image during training.

Although it has to be said that the above research was carried out on learners not involved in a Project 2000-type course, it is nevertheless in keeping with earlier studies, and could perhaps give us a preventative framework around which we can build mentor development.

The student self-image appears to play a crucial part in determining how they react, not only with regard to leaving, but also in relation to the effectiveness of education. Bradby (1989) noted that there was a relationship between those students with a low self-esteem and a higher level of anxiety. It appeared that those falling into this group were particularly vulnerable and were most likely, along with those at the other extreme (very high self-esteem/low anxiety) to leave.

McGouran (1991) threw some light on how the above effects may be compounded by the reactions of qualified staff to changes in the curriculum. Broadly the study highlighted, for the purposes of our discussion, four major areas of concern:

1. Allocation of time to supervise and teach students.
2. Students' lack of practical ability.
3. Students' lack of knowledge of anatomy and physiology.
4. Difficulty in implementing the mentorship system.

It would appear, therefore, that the difficulties which lead to possible breakdown in both learner and qualified staff satisfaction and effectiveness of the education process in the clinical area are numerous.

# The counselling role of the mentor

Having explored the areas of student and mentor satisfaction (or otherwise), this section will help the mentor to explore some ways of overcoming some of these problems.

The subject of communication has been covered in earlier chapters but it would seem appropriate to examine one special aspect, namely the counselling role of the mentor. Perhaps the best place to start is to examine the concept of dependent and helping behaviour.

## Helping behaviour

One aspect of behaviour familiar to health care professionals in their day-to-day activities is that of "care-giving" (nurture) which, along with "care-seeking" are the most common types of pro-social behaviour. In terms of the mentor–student relationship, both the ability to recognise dependent behaviour and to offer the best possible help to the student or colleague in question are essential.

Most of us are more than capable of recognising when a physical need requires our intervention (such as illness), and at times emotional needs (such as bereavement) may have their own prescribed course of action such as compassionate leave. An integral part of the mentor's role is to ensure, as far as possible, the students well-being in relation to the other areas of dependent and nurturing behaviours.

## Dependency and nurture

Care-seeking behaviour (dependency) may be a means for the individual to attain something (such as comfort, relief from physical illness and sometimes building of self-esteem) which may not be achieved independently for one reason or another (*instrumental dependency*), although it may also be sought for purely pleasurable ends (*emotional dependency*). Instrumental dependency can be illustrated by the student attempting a new skill and asking for your support/guidance, while emotional dependency is demonstrated by the student who, although competent in an area of practice, still seeks your help in order to gain praise and attention. This second example may be indicative of the student who has a lack of self-esteem.

Generally, with a few notable exceptions such as losing a job or bereavement, emotional dependency is less tolerated by society, although instrumental dependence continues to be socially acceptable, probably due to the inevitability of a loss of independence at some time during our lives through illness, disability or, conceivably, going through a more formal learning experience such as in education. It is interesting to note (Baker, 1990) that some students attach great importance to the counselling role of the mentor, hence underlining the relevance of the dependency relationship.

Perhaps one of the most obvious areas in education where emotional dependency occurs is where a student fails an assessment and needs the support of the mentor and possibly others, including personal tutor, friends and colleagues. Such an event will naturally lead to a sharp decline in self-esteem in most individuals. It would be a mistake to assume that most of us could "pick ourselves up and dust ourselves down" immediately after such an event. A problem does arise, however, in deciding how best to help the student, but perhaps a bigger problem is recognising the type of support they require. It seems that there is a process which we need to work through in order to reach a decision to help someone and that sometimes even with the most blatant evidence to the contrary, we proffer little or no help at all (Darley and Latane, 1968).

## Altruism

*Altruism* refers to rendering help to other persons without thought of personal gain or reward. It is arguably a trait that we would all like to think that we possess although it has been shown that it is not quite as straightforward as it at first appears. The emergence of altruistic behaviour is covered elsewhere (Oliver, 1993) but for the purposes of our discussion, we will concentrate on some of the decisions which may have to be reached by the onlooker or "by-stander" in order that help may be given.

### The bystander effect

In real-life situations, even those where there is a risk of death to the victim (Darley and Latane, 1968), help is rendered usually when the following processes have been worked through.

## Noticing the emergency

It seems obvious to state that we have to notice an event before we act upon it, although several factors may prevent this from happening:

1. We did not physically perceive it.
2. We may have been preoccupied.
3. Others around us lead us to define the situation wrongly by their attitudes or actions.

## Interpreting the situation

1. Usually determined by a group of people such as a ward team. (What constitutes an emergency?)
2. Finding an alternative/wrong interpretation, e.g. assuming the student is unhappy or distressed for a reason other than the real one.

## The decision to intervene

1. Naturally dependent on the previous stage.
2. Decisions regarding whether it is our responsibility are made.
3. There may be "diffused responsibility", in other words, we may have assumed that someone else was going to do something or that somebody else should take the responsibility.
4. We assess the amount of physical or emotional safety involved to us.
5. We may even consider what personal gain is involved.

## Listening skills

It makes sense to say that if we are going to identify an individual's difficulties we need to be able to listen effectively. The reader is referred to the discussion and activities in Chapter one.

For a more complete account of the practical aspects of the counselling role, the reader is referred to Tschudin (1991).

# Guiding

As stated earlier, the role of the mentor is multifaceted and it should not be assumed that it is purely, or in any way exclusively, a counselling relationship; more active intervention is often required. The mentoree in a strange environment will need some form of orientation to local values and, for want of a better word, customs, in order to be able to function in the organisation. This is particularly the case when placed in an environment which is more specialised in nature than they are used to, e.g. from general surgery to paediatrics.

Socialisation in the area is essential if the mentoree is to form meaningful relationships within both the social and educational contexts.

# Advising

Perhaps in contrast to the counselling role of the mentor is that of adviser. The mentor is inevitably viewed as a member of staff who is experienced both clinically and in terms of providing support for students and as such is in an ideal position to advise both at career and social levels (Zey, 1984). It should be remembered that the student is confronted within a short space of time with numerous, highly varied experiences which may invariably at times lie outside their expectations. This may naturally involve the student in having to deal with inner conflicts as to choice of career and how to deal with clinical situations on a day-to-day basis. It is important that the mentor is able to help them to deal with this situation both on a global and day-to-day basis, in other words to help them put things into perspective.

The role of adviser is obviously not as clear-cut as it may at first seem. In terms of dealing with a dying patient, the role of adviser is frequently paired with that of counsellor, and indeed it could be said that where any situation arises in which personal emotions and professional duty are involved, then these two components of the role may be inextricably linked. In terms of the learning outcomes that the mentoree is working towards, then the advising role, depending as it does on the experience of the mentor, tends to be more clear-cut. Even in this instance it is difficult to divide the two completely with listening skills being a vital component of both.

In examining the role of mentor, certain key aspects have been examined and the assumption has been made that the mentor is not involved in formal supervision or assessment. It has been discussed earlier that this is sometimes difficult to achieve. In other words, it is very difficult to be both the student's assessor and guide simultaneously.

It is now appropriate to discuss the role of the preceptor in order to complete the picture of providing support for the student and newly qualified staff nurse in the learning environment.

# Preceptorship

The role of the *preceptor* has gained prominence in recent years in two major areas of nursing. Firstly, preceptorship is seen as a partner to the mentor role, indeed it completes the other half of the equation for a student in terms of assessing and supervising. Secondly (UKCC, 1993), the role of the preceptor is identified as vital to the development of the support of newly registered practitioners.

Possibly the simplest definition of preceptor is that of a teacher or instructor, although the role is far more involved than this would suggest. Lee (1991) suggests that the preceptor role is "probably more of a combination of the roles of mentor, supervisor and assessor". It is probably quite correct to assume that the roles of mentor and preceptor are indivisible in some areas particularly when referring to the preceptor's role in relation to newly qualified staff. For the purposes of this discussion however, the preceptor's role will be examined in terms of its socialisation, facilitation and assessing components especially.

## Socialisation – a role of preceptors or mentors

In a review of the literature (Goldenburg, 1993; Iwasiw, 1993) professional socialisation

> is seen as a specific portion of adult socialisation, a complex interactive process by which the content of the professional role (skills, knowledge and behaviour) is learned, and the values, attitudes and goals integral to the profession and sense of occupational identity which are characteristic of a member of that profession are internalised.

Viewed in this way, namely as socialisation being a key role of the preceptor, the role of preceptor is described by Goldenburg and Iwasiw as "an intense, one-to-one reality-based, clinical learning experience between an accomplished staff nurse and a neophyte".

It can be seen that the role of mentor and that of preceptor according this predominantly American/Canadian definition are to a large extent combined when comparing it with earlier definitions given by the ENB and UKCC.

## The preceptor and facilitating learning

The skills of a teacher are discussed elsewhere in the text, and are of course vital attributes of the effective preceptor. Facilitation on the other hand (Brown, 1989) is viewed as the process of enabling another person to achieve goals. This can equally be applied to the student, newly qualified staff member or health care assistant undertaking a National Vocational Qualification (NVQ).

Craddock (1993) emphasises that "the route to confidence in which knowledge, experience and performing nursing acts are integrated is via facilitation". Brown (1989) goes on to point out that certain key factors are essential for effective facilitation and hence some responsibility for the following factors must be assumed by the preceptor.

1. *Task*: assessing; planning; implementing; evaluation of care.
2. *Needs of the learner*: learning style; previous experience; interest.
3. *Skills of the Facilitator*: knowledge base; motivation; competence.

Briggs (1985) found that trained staff sometimes used students as a source of information and viewed them as being more up to date. If this is still the case with current nursing curricula, then this will dramatically reduce the effectiveness of the role of the preceptor especially in terms of Brown's views on the facilitation of learning. The implications for the student of perceiving that their preceptor has less knowledge than they do may not altogether be a disadvantage if viewed from the standpoint of socialisation where both the preceptor (socialiser) and the individual joining the group are mutually influenced (Hurley-Wilson, 1988).

If we return to the definition given earlier (Goldenburg, 1993; Iwasiw, 1993) it can be gleaned that by virtue of the intense one-to-one relationship established, deficiencies of knowledge on either side will inevitably become apparent. It would clearly be unacceptable, despite all that has been said above, for the preceptor to be seen as clinically incompetent, although at the same time it should be viewed that the student will inevitably bring not only their own personal experiences to the learning situation, but also may be able to supplement the preceptor's knowledge, particularly within the realms of social sciences.

It has been clearly identified earlier that part of the role of the preceptor is that of teaching and assessing, and the reader is referred to the relevant chapters in the text.

## Supporting the preceptor/mentor

The role of preceptor/mentor can be a stressful one and thought needs to be given in any organisation to the support that will be necessary to help individuals perform this role. Some specialist departments, e.g. care of the elderly units, have established preceptor/mentor support groups. These groups meet regularly to discuss the role as well as any difficulties that have been experienced. This would seem to be one useful approach but the role of the ward or unit manager in providing support must not be forgotten.

## Conclusions

The roles of mentor and preceptor have been discussed in terms of both their uniqueness and commonalities. It can be seen that particularly where relationships are considered, the distinction between the two roles is difficult to define. At the same time, the assessing component of the preceptor's role in particular may render the role incompatible with the notion of combining it with a mentorship component. The commonly accepted idea that a mentor should be chosen by the student may also be at variance with the concept that the preceptor should have considerable clinical experience in order to carry out the role effectively.

The distinction between the two roles is perhaps easier to achieve in the pre-registration domain rather than with newly qualified staff where the mentor and preceptorship roles may be more easily combined; particularly when considering the high degree of socialisation content involved with a member of staff working permanently in the area.

On a practical level the availability of enough staff to provide both a preceptor and a mentor for each student cannot be ignored and it seems likely that this should emerge as the most likely reason for the roles being combined in some areas despite advice to the contrary (ENB, 1989). Various permutations may be tried in order to overcome this problem, especially by introducing a dual role whereby a member of staff may act as a preceptor for one individual but as a mentor for another. Alternatively, a small group of staff could be identified as preceptors (perhaps those with most clinical expertise), whereas others could be regarded solely as mentors. Whatever the arrangement, an organising/arbitration role must be assumed by the individual in order to ensure the smooth running of the system and also to intervene in situations where support is required by either the student or mentor/preceptor.

# Summary

As far as the English National Board (89)17 is concerned, a mentor is

A person selected by the student to assist, befriend, guide, advise and counsel (but who would not normally be involved in the formal supervision or assessment of that particular student) (ENB, 1989).

Anforth (1992) in reviewing the literature e.g. (Barlow, 1991; Burnard, 1990) is concerned that the role of mentor still requires further definition or as Haggerty (1986) maintains it is still a "definition quagmire".

Certainly in the past (e.g. Lee, 1991) the role of mentor and assessor were sometimes combined and this naturally would effect the nature of the relationship.

An essentially non-threatening relationship is essential in order that the essence of the mentoring expectations is not damaged (ENB, 1989).

One of the roles of the mentor, by virtue of the relationship which has been built up, is to recognise the effect that stress is having on their mentoree.

The student's self-image appears to play a crucial part in determining how they react, not only with regard to leaving, but also in relation to the effectiveness of education.

An integral part of the mentor's role is to ensure, as far as possible, the student's well-being in relation to the other areas of dependent and nurturing behaviours.

Care-seeking behaviour (dependency) may be a means for the individual to attain something (such as comfort, relief of physical illness and sometimes building of self-esteem).

The mentoree in a strange environment will need some form of orientation to local values and, for want of a better word, customs, in order to be able to function in the organisation.

The mentor is inevitably viewed as a member of staff who is experienced both clinically and in terms of providing support for students and as such is in an ideal position to advise both at career and social levels (Zey, 1984).

Preceptorship is seen as a partner to the mentor role, indeed it completes the other half of the equation for a student in terms of assessing and supervising.

The role of the preceptor is identified as vital to the development of the support of newly registered practitioners (UKCC, 1990).

The role of preceptor is described by Goldenburg (1993) and Iwasiw (1993) as "an intense, one-to-one reality-based, clinical learning experience between an accomplished staff nurse and a neophyte".

Brown (1989) views facilitation as the process of enabling another person to achieve goals. Craddock (1993) emphasises that "the route to confidence in which knowledge, experience and performing nursing acts are integrated is via facilitation".

The role of preceptor/mentor can be a stressful one and thought needs to be given in any organisation to the support that will be necessary to help individuals perform this role.

# Related activities

## Activity 1

Set up a discussion group with colleagues who are also mentors and attempt to establish the following:

1. What type of mentor do they perceive themselves to be?
2. How do they describe their role?
3. Are their roles prescribed or are they chosen by the student?

## Activity 2

Set up a discussion group with students who are gaining experience in your area and attempt to establish the following:

1. What type of mentor do they perceive themselves as having?
2. How do they describe the role of their mentor?
3. Were they allocated a mentor or did they have any choice?

Briefly record your findings from activities 1 and 2 (approximately 500 words).

## Activity 3

Using the discussion group from activities 1 and 2 produce a list of aspects of your role including the following

1. Those aspects that you perceive the students find helpful.
2. Those aspects that you have difficulty with and that you perceive the student finds unhelpful.

Ask your student(s) to complete a similar exercise and then compare the two lists in a free-ranging discussion. Briefly record your findings (approximately 500 words) (see Chapter 5).

## Activity 4

An advocate is a person who speaks or acts on behalf of another. In your role as mentor, there will be occasions when you will act as the students' advocate. While it should be remembered that it is your role also to encourage independence, there will be occasions when you will need to intervene.

What signs would lead you to suspect that the student was experiencing personal difficulties?

## Activity 5

To what extent can objectivity be maintained by an individual involved in facilitating the socialisation of a student/newly qualified member of staff as well as the assessment of their perfomance? (Can the mentor/preceptor role be combined?) Make short notes.

## Activity 6

1. What would you hope to gain from setting up a preceptor/mentor support group? (Discuss with your colleagues.)
2. Based on the above perceptions, write terms of reference for this group.
3. Identify key personnel who may act in a supporting role to the group (managers, tutors, etc.).

## References

Anforth, P. (1992) Mentors not assessors. *Nurse Education Today*, **12**, 299–302.

Baker, S. (1990) The key to nurse education? *Nursing Standard* **4**, 39–43.

Barlow, S. (1991) Impossible dream . . . mentorship in UK nurse education. *Nursing Times*, **87**, 53–54.

Bradby, M. (1990) Status passage into nursing: another view of the process of socialization into nursing. *Journal of Advanced Nursing*, **15**, 1220–1225.

Briggs, K. (1985) Group facilitation skills: how can they be learned. *Nurse Education Today*, **5**(4), 143–146.

Brown, H. (1989) Facilitation strategies – the key to developing clinical excellence. In P. Bradshaw (ed.) *Teaching and Assessing in the Clinical Nursing Practice*. Herts: Prentice Hall International.

Burnard, P. (1990) The student experience: adult learning and mentoring revisited. *Nurse Education Today*, **10**(5) 349–354.

Craddock, E. (1993) Developing the facilitator role in the clinical area. *Nurse Education Today*, **13**, 217–224.

Darley, J.M. and Latane, B. (1968) Bystander intervention in emergencies: diffusion of responsibility. *Journal of Personality and Social Psychology*, **8**, 377–383.

ENB (1989) *Preparation of Teachers, Practitioners/ Teachers Mentors and Supervisers in the Context of Project 2000*. London: ENB.

Fogg, D.J. (1989) A study of wastage in nurse education: no way to treat a lady or man. Unpublished Thesis, School of Education, University of East Anglia.

Goldenberg, D. (1993) Professional Socialisation of Nursing

Haggerty, B. (1986) A second look at mentors. *Nursing Outlook*, **34**(1), 16–24.

Hurley-Wilson, B. (1988) Socialisation for roles. In M.E. Hardy and M.E. Conway (eds) *Role Theory. Perspectives for Health Professionals*, 2nd edn. Connecticut: Appleton & Lange.

Iwasiw, C. (1993) Students as an outcome of a senior clinical preceptorship experience. *Nurse Education Today*, **13**, 3–15.

Lee, S.J. (1991) Guidelines for the role of preceptor. *Nursing Standard*, **6**(6), 28–30.

Levinson, D.J. *et al.* (1978) *The Seasons of a Man's Life*. New York: A.A. Knopf.

McGouran, V.E. (1991) Qualified nurses' response to change. A study of the response of clinical staff to alteration in the pre-registration curriculum. Unpublished Thesis, UEA.

Morle, K.M.F. (1990) Mentorship – is it a case of the emperor's new clothes or a rose by any other name. *Nurse Education Today*, **10**(1), 66–69.

Oliver, R.W. (1993) *Psychology and Health Care*. London: Ballière Tindall.

Palmer, E.A. (1987) A study to introduce mentoring in nursing. Unpublished Thesis, South Bank Polytechnic.

Tschudin, V. (1991) *Counselling for Nurses*. London: Ballière Tindall.

UKCC (1993) *The Council's proposed Standards for Post Registration Education*. London: UKCC.

Zey, M.C. (1984) *The Mentor Connection*. Dow Jones.

# chapter five

# Learning theories

## Introduction

It is very tempting when preparing a text which is aimed at the practical considerations of preceptorship to find a case for omitting a traditional approach of presenting learning theories. It is sometimes difficult to put over the work which is essential to each theory, whilst at the same time maintaining its practical application. It is in fact a waste of time if such theories cannot be applied to education in the clinical area. However, all of the major theories of learning, although they originate from different schools of thought and by implication will advocate different teaching strategies, nevertheless have their place, principally because we cannot define any form of nurse education as being the sole province of any one school of thought.

Various questions underlie the basis of this chapter and it has been organised in such a way as to provide some practical answers. For example, is the learning that takes place for a resuscitation procedure necessarily the same as that which will help us deal with the bereaved? Is the learning which occurs during social science education necessarily the same as that which will occur during the study of biological sciences? Many of the theorists mentioned below have argued, sometimes convincingly, that their theories can be applied to any subject and it appears that the debate here is mainly centred upon the context in which the subject is taught (i.e. in the clinical situation) rather than the subject matter itself. For these reasons as well as for convenience of the reader, this chapter is organised in a way which departs from the traditional approaches which examine each school of thought in isolation, and looks at the context in which they are applied.

One of the major areas which is continually debated in education is quite how individual learning can be, and further, how experience can contribute to the learning process. There are, quite naturally, those who are for and against this humanistic approach to education. Many have argued with some justification that whereas every individual is different, we nevertheless have to work, at least to some extent, to a preset curriculum and meet the criteria of a preset assessment strategy. The alternative argument is therefore discussed in relation to the behaviourist viewpoint which takes into account the educator being able to predict what the student will learn in response to a given situation. The arguments for each continue to rage in education circles, but it should be said here that the authors are expressing no preference for either, whilst at the same time appreciating the merits and disadvantages of each.

A slightly less contentious issue concerns the nature of concept formation and problem solving, but once again, purists will argue the merits of one school of thought or another. The cognitive theorists, on the one hand, describe a process by which problem solving can be achieved through education, whereas those advocating a gestalt approach place far more emphasis on the way in which information is presented. Once again, as with the previous instance, there does not appear to be a coherent reason why both arguments should not carry equal weight and be incorporated into teaching strategies successfully.

It is of course up to the reader quite how they use the information contained in this chapter, although it is intended to give them enough information to be able to examine their learning environment, the subject matter in hand and the outcomes they hope to achieve and then to be selective in the direction of their teaching.

It seems logical that the discussion should start with the person who is at the centre of the education process, namely the individual student.

# The individual, experience and learning

The humanistic school of psychology is certainly not new, although the concepts that underpin it are still a matter of much debate in education. The underlying premise that each one of us is an individual who cannot have their behaviour predicted in any given situation is a difficult one to grasp because in its extreme form the implications are that we can never be sure that anyone will learn from any situation, thus preventing any tangible use of predetermined learning outcomes.

One of the earliest humanistic psychologists is Maslow, whose work (discussed in earlier chapters), though possibly the oldest, is still used as a framework for both nursing care (e.g. Roper *et al.*, 1981) and education. For the purposes of our discussion, we will look at the theory of self-actualisation mainly from the viewpoint of Rogers (1969).

# Rogerian perspectives on education

Out of all of the humanistic psychologists, Rogers is possibly the most emphatic that one individual can never be totally understood by another. In order to arrive at this conclusion, Rogers makes several observations which have an enormous implication for the learning environment.

Rogers uses as the basis of his theory the fact that we all have a need for *positive regard*, in other words, we all need to feel good about ourselves. The ways in which we achieve such positive regard are naturally dependent, to some extent, on the reactions of other people to our actions. Put another way, do we do things that will please others, but may be against our true feelings? This is the case not only in childhood, but also happens during the course of our working lives and education.

Feeling positive regard as a result of what other people want or expect us to do leads to what Rogers terms *conditional positive regard* namely, positive regard which is conditioned by other people's reactions and approval. In education terms it could be said that somebody achieves conditional positive regard if in completing an assessment that they had no desire to complete they achieve a pass grade. If on the other hand we have positive regard despite what anybody thinks of us, we have *unconditional positive regard*, in other words, we feel valued by others even if we do not live up to their expectations.

It follows logically that if, as Rogers says, we exist substantially with conditional positive regard, we are operating to standards that we perceive, either rightly or wrongly, other people wish us to achieve. These are known as *conditions of worth* and are readily observable within the nurse education setting. Conditions of worth may take the form of professional behaviour, academic standards, achieving learning outcomes and even holding certain attitudes and values.

Eventually we will internalise these conditions so that we may behave and achieve in a way prescribed by the group or society in which we are operating and hence will gain the approval (or rather avoid disapproval) of others. Rogers terms this *positive self-regard* and it is antagonistic to the individual reaching true self-actualisation. The reasons for this are immediately obvious in as much as if the individual cannot achieve growth without the restraints placed on them by others, then they will never reach their full potential, but will rather reach the potential approved of by others. Feeling good about ourselves for whatever reason, is of course by any other name, achieving positive self-esteem, and this is a major landmark that the individual strives to achieve and will often go to great lengths to maintain it. Because positive self-regard is self-esteem achieved through fulfilling the conditions placed on us by others, Rogers sees this as potentially damaging.

In order to achieve true self-actualisation, Rogers advocates helping the individual to achieve *unconditional self-regard*. This he does because of his belief that the incompatibility of an individual's true feelings with those of the conditions of worth placed on them is a major source of maladjustment. Although unconditional positive self-regard may possibly be achieved in small areas of an individual's life, it is difficult to conceptualise how this may be achieved in a more generalised sense, for to do so could be at the expense of the individual's standing in a group or society.

In its pure form, as with many other theories, the Rogerian concept of education, namely learning which fulfils totally the individual's need and does not place restraints upon them seems impossible to achieve within nurse education.

## Applications of Rogerian theory to clinical education

No matter how much we may agree or disagree, getting a nursing qualification has a significant emphasis on achieving an end product which by its very definition means meeting standards laid down by others. This is not to say, however, that the process by which we achieve this end cannot, at least in part, have a humanistic orientation. Teaching strategies are discussed elsewhere in the text but, it is worthwhile at this juncture to list some of those which may illustrate individual learning.

1. *Unconditional positive regard*. This may in part be achieved by the use of negotiating, learning contracts with the student, individual tutorials, pastoral support, buzz groups, brainstorming.
2. *Conditional positive regard*. Attempting to achieve behavioural objectives, completing assessments, formal teaching methods, may all lead to the conditions of others being placed on the individual.
3. *Positive self-regard*. The acquisition of group values either from influential individuals or from the expectations and rules of societies/organisations.
4. *Unconditional positive self-regard*. This may be achieved with entirely self-initiated learning with no perceivable outside influences. Although virtually impossible to achieve, it seems most likely that those undertaking self-financed open learning courses can go at least some way to achieving this.

It is not simply the case that a particular method will lead to any one of the above outcomes although the method chosen will have an effect. For instance, participating in a discussion group, may for some individuals lead to unconditional positive regard whereas for others it may lead to positive self-regard, depending on the subject in hand and those people present in the group.

Rogers (1969) places significant emphasis on the student-centred learning approach and as such advocates those methods which allow individuals to express themselves freely, and possibly most importantly for our discussion, he emphasises the essential nature of "doing", rather than sitting down and learning. More especially, it is perhaps relevant to consider this in terms of the student's supernumerary status and to reiterate the unsatisfactory status of purely non-participative observation visits for the majority of the time.

The role played by experiential learning is a corner-stone of Rogers' theory and is also the basis of a more practical application of humanistic psychology, namely that expounded by Kolb (1984).

# Experiential learning theory

Kolb (1984) views learning as a lifelong event and sees knowledge as emerging through the transformation of experience. Kolb, following extensive research, suggested that individuals whose learning styles did not match the environment in which they were learning were less satisfied and felt more alienated than those whose learning styles matched their environment.

Generally speaking, experiential learning theory can be described as a cyclical learning process in which Kolb describes four types of learning competencies

1. Feeling (concrete experience competencies).
2. Perceiving (reflective observation competencies).
3. Thinking (abstract conceptualisation competencies).
4. Behaving (active experimentation competencies).

The learning process cycle in its broadest terms could be said to comprise the individual experiencing an actual situation, perceiving it from different angles, reflecting on its significance, forming theories about what is happening and finally testing those theories out in practice.

Naturally, we are not all as good at some parts of the learning process as we are at others and our past experiences may, for instance, enable us to be rather better at being able to reflect on a situation than to form theories about it. This will be dependent on how the individual has developed through life and their past experiences. It should be re-emphasised that this is a cyclical learning process and that all of what Kolb terms as competencies need to be used. It should come as no surprise, however, that each one of these competencies requires rather a different learning style and since we are better at some competencies than others, the results of Kolb's research reveals that individuals will have predominantly one learning style in preference to others.

As stated earlier, dissatisfaction will occur if the learning style imposed on the individual is incompatible with the competency that they favour and it is appropriate at this juncture to examine briefly quite what these styles are, and loosely which competencies they are compatible with. Figure 5.1 represents diagrammatically the learning cycle and the learning styles.

If we use Kolb's own definition of learning styles as being a way of processing information, it makes sense to complete the equation and to examine which situations and teaching strategies would be compatible with each individual. Laschinger (1990) in reviewing Kolb's theory summarises learning styles which are most appropriate to the competencies.

Those with strong concrete experience and reflective observation skills (*divergers*) prefer concrete experiences as distinct from theoretical ones and tend to be more person orientated. Those with strong concrete experience and active experimentation skills (*accommodators*), will be better at carrying out practical plans and at the same time will also seek out new experiences. At the same time, these individuals will tend not to be particularly analytical and may be more instinctive in their actions. Those with highly developed abstract conceptualisation and reflective observation competencies (*assimilators*) tend to be rather better at forming concepts

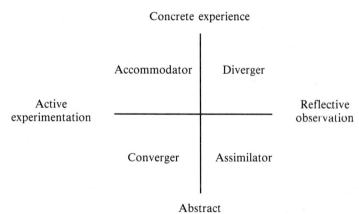

Concrete experience

Accommodator    Diverger

Active
experimentation                                    Reflective
observation

Converger    Assimilator

Abstract
conceptualisation

**Figure 5.1.** Learning cycle and learning styles (Kolb, 1976).

through experiences. Those with strong abstract conceptualisation and active experimentation skills (*convergers*) tend to exhibit skill in problem solving, particularly where a single answer is sought.

It should be remembered that although Kolb's theory gives us considerable insight into the differing learning styles of the individuals, it can only be used effectively if the individuals involved have been appropriately tested (Kolb, 1976; Kolb and Wolfe, 1981) to determine which competencies they excel in. Conversely, most individuals may be able to identify their own particular strengths and weaknesses and hence their most effective learning style.

The theories discussed so far can now perhaps be seen in a different light, in as much as it is ill-advised to make assumptions that all individuals will process information in an identical way in response to poorly selected teaching strategies which have not taken into account the diversity of learning styles that they may possess.

## Achievement of predetermined learning outcomes

The behaviourist school of thought is prominent in theories of learning and was typified by Bloom (1956) in terms of education. It is perhaps unfashionable to consider a subject such as nursing as producing practitioners who will achieve predetermined outcomes rather than a diversity of perspectives and knowledge gained through experience. In many ways the behaviourist approach is far removed from, and even directly opposed to, the humanistic approach to education and it could be said that it only really has one thing in common with it, namely, that used in its extreme form, it is virtually unworkable. The originator of behaviourism, Watson, was at pains to point out that only observable behaviours should be examined rather than surmising about the mental mechanisms that were taking place. This gained great prominence in the early part of the century.

The situation in clinical education on first inspection is not behaviourist in the overall context but it can be seen by the examples given below that some learning experiences may be most appropriately explained using this approach. The theories of Pavlov seem most unlikely to fall under even this category but it is arguable that this type of learning in some situations forms the basis of higher forms of learning at a later stage. This is further expounded by Gagne (1974), whose work will be discussed later in the chapter.

## Classical conditioning

The reflexes that Pavlov described were of two types, unconditioned and conditioned. **Unconditioned reflexes** (UCR) are innate, and include such basic functions as salivation. **Conditioned reflexes** (CR) are formed as a result of experience. The UCR is the normal response to an **unconditioned stimulus** (UCS) such as food. A conditioned stimulus (CS) is a previously neutral item which, through "pairing" with a UCS, produces a new response. An example which could perhaps clarify the picture can be seen in a nurse's response to a cardiac arrest. Before training, the nurse's response to an individual who has collapsed (UCS) could be a sudden release of adrenalin with all of its effects (UCR). Through training, the nurse can be taught to examine the patient's pulse, which if absent (CS), may elicit behaviours such as lying the patient flat, inserting an artificial airway, etc. (CR). It may be the case that the nurse has gleaned that asystole being recorded on the cardiac monitor is a sign of cardiac arrest, and this, if paired with a collapsed patient, may also act as a CS, and instigate the appropriate responses, if paired on several occasions. If, however, the nurse is confronted with an asystole trace due to the monitor being disconnected, eventually the CR will be "extinguished". The reflex can be regained by finding a new CS, in this case the one that should have been used in the first place, namely the pulse. This is known as "disinhibition". As the training progresses, the nurse will begin to "generalise" the CR to a variety of situations, rather than just a patient on a coronary care unit.

## Operant conditioning

From numerous well-documented experiments in operant conditioning, in both animals and humans, Skinner (1938) proposed that the following factors should be present before learning can take place.

1. Each step of the learning process must be short and should grow out of previous learned behaviour.
2. In the early stages learning should be regularly rewarded and at all stages be carefully controlled by a schedule of continuous or intermittent *reinforcement*. This reinforcement is a feature of discovery learning in as much as reinforcement for students is a discovery of a concept by its own efforts. For instance, if students are given anti-a and anti-b antigen solutions they may work out for themselves which blood group they belong to.
3. Reward should follow quickly when a correct response appears. This is referred to as feedback and is based on the principle that motivation is enhanced when we are informed of our progress. Laboratory experiments provide such feedback. With careful explanation and supervision, the student will usually be able to achieve a predicted outcome.
4. The learner should be given an opportunity to discover stimulus discrimination for the most likely path to success.

It could be argued that all of learning can be explained in terms of operant conditioning as long as interpretation of positive reinforcement can be widened sufficiently to account for the diversity of situations that the learner may find themselves in. Certainly the immediate feedback from academic work is an obvious example but in the clinical area, more diverse reinforcers need to be identified. For example, in order for positive reinforcement to take place, the learner will have had to have done something in order for it to be reinforced such as improvement in a patient's condition or praise from their preceptor.

From these principles Skinner devised a scheme known as "Programmed Learning", now extensively employed using computer-assisted learning techniques, so that each student may progress at their own pace. Like discovery learning, however, the method is a relatively slow one, particularly in terms of preparation time for the teacher or instructor. It is of particular value with students of mixed ability and/or when a subject area is particularly difficult.

It is now more common practice, with the exception of programmed learning mentioned above, to use a behaviourist approach in the more basic skills training such as cardiac arrest procedures, although it should be mentioned that over a period of time problem-solving behaviour should develop.

# Types of learning (Gagne's)

Gagne's theory of learning has a strong behavioural slant and, unlike Kolb, describes the learning process in terms of a hierarchy as distinct from a cycle. Behaviour according to Gagne (1975) should be compared before and after the learning situation to determine whether learning has taken place, and hence Gagne's interpretation of learning goes along the lines of the earlier behaviourists in as far as he defines it as a change in behaviour.

It has been discussed earlier in the chapter that nurse education is highly dependent in some areas on a product approach, in other words we need to be able to predict to an extent how much learning has taken place in order to ascertain whether an individual has attained a certain standard. The systematic approach that Gagne utilises may correlate well with aspects of the curriculum such as the nursing process (Condell and Elliott, 1989). In terms of more lateral thinking he can be seen as equally incompatible, in particular where problem solving utilising past experience is involved. Gagne advocates a teacher-centred approach by virtue of the fact that although he regards the student as having capabilities which are internal to them, the stimulation is nevertheless outside the learner (Gagne, 1985).

The hierarchy of learning is briefly described below and it will be noticed that at least up to the chaining level and possibly as far as multiple discrimination there are strong implications for psychomotor skills learning (Coulter, 1990).

## Gagne's hierarchy of learning

1. *Signal learning*. This is equivalent to Pavlov's Conditioned Response.
2. *Stimulus–response learning*. This is equivalent to Skinner's Discriminated Operant Conditioning.
3. *Chaining*. A chain of two or more stimulus–response connections achieved by learning stimulus–response connections, carrying out the steps in the chain in a set sequence, carrying out all elements of the chain close together and repeating the performance to provide reinforcement.
4. *Verbal association*. Learning verbal chains.
5. *Multiple discrimination*. Learning to discriminate between stimuli which resemble each other.
6. *Concept learning*. Learning to make a common response to stimuli that can be organised into a class of objects rather than an individual example, with each component of the class sharing common characteristics.

7. *Principle learning*. A chain of two or more concepts.
8. *Problem solving*. Solving problems by the use of principles.

As a consequence of Gagne's assertion that the learning process focuses heavily on teacher-centred approaches, great emphasis is placed on how information is presented. From the behaviourist's point of view, this can be translated into how the stimulus is presented. This does not mean that the internal conditions of learning such as the student's capabilities are not important, indeed they are crucial. Methods of presenting material are covered elsewhere in the text but it should be mentioned here that Gagne's ideas on stimulus presentation and optimising learner's capabilities range from those factors which will gain the student's attention and facilitate recall, to presenting the actual stimulus/information and being able to facilitate information retention.

# Building concepts and problem solving

## Gestalt approaches

In Chapter four, Gestalt theory was explored briefly in terms of the psychological organisation of material. Here some concrete examples of its utilisation are discussed.

The Gestalt school would be in agreement with Gagne about the importance of presenting material but would most certainly be in opposition to the behavioural slant which underlies his theory. Gestalt (insightful learning) relies heavily on the individual being able to arrive at solutions as a result of being given information which they will then organise into a complete picture.

There are many occasions where adequate preparation is just not feasible, for instance, when an impromptu teaching session evolves from the admission of a new patient. However, by utilising Gestalt psychology which is concerned with organised forms and patterns in human perception, thinking and learning (Curzon, 1990), we will aid the student's learning process. Briefly, it can be applied as follows:

1. *Symmetry* – in other words the session should be divided into an introduction, development and conclusion. This stage, as with some others, is highly dependent on the student's previous knowledge.
2. *Contiguity* – ensure that any reinforcements, such as relevant observations on the patient, pieces of equipment, etc., are shown either at the time of the session or as soon as possible.
3. *Similarity* – try not to "jump" from subject to subject within the same session. If this is not possible, at least ensure that similarity is created by referring subjects back to a focal point. For instance, if the care of a patient is being discussed, and a diversion is needed to talk about the actions of certain drugs, then this will need to be individualized to the patient.
4. *Closure* – try to plan the session in such a way as to allow the student to complete some parts for themselves. This can be done in at least two ways. Firstly, it can be achieved by the use of questions, e.g. "so, if Mr Jones is retaining large amounts of sodium, what would you look for?" Naturally, care should be taken not to demotivate the student by making them feel threatened. Secondly, the student can be given something to observe or further research, but if this is done, then time needs to be put aside later to discuss their findings so that it can be integrated into the overall subject.

For a pictorial interpretation of Gestalt approaches, the reader is directed to Chapter four.

# Discovery learning

It could be argued that more traditional forms of learning theory such as the behavioural theories place an emphasis on the information being presented to the student and then practical experience given in order that they may apply it (see also assimilation theory below). An alternative theory which runs contrary to this approach is discovery learning (Bruner, 1960), which is essentially a student-centred approach which assumes that knowledge will be internalised as a result of experimentation and experience.

Essentially, discovery learning is concerned with the development of concepts from processes which have enabled the individual to find common properties in objects or situations which will enable them to classify them into groups and to be able to apply general rules to them. Naturally, this process is a continual evolution and cannot be looked at as an isolated event as the student will continue to evaluate new experiences within the context of earlier concepts which have been formed. The logical consequence of this in terms of education is that the student will be able to revisit concepts throughout a course of study and to expand them in the light of new experience (spiral curriculum). The process of discovery, although quite a complex phenomenon, can be divided into two major activities with evaluation of what is happening occurring as an on-going feature:

1. *Induction* – (taking particular instances and using them to devise a general case) with a minimum of instruction.
2. *Errorful learning* – employing trial and error strategies in which there is a high probability of errors and mistakes before an acceptable generalisation is possible.

It could be argued that in terms of everyday life, discovery learning occurs naturally and is effective in helping us develop. In terms of more formal education its uses have also been advocated, but at times with reservations (Cronbach, 1966), in as much as its function is sometimes seen as specialised and limited, although at the same time it could increase motivation, resourcefulness and satisfaction.

The use of discovery appears to be centred upon certain conditions all of which may be decisions which a ward-based facilitator may be able to have some influence over. For example, in terms of the experience being process or product based, will the preceptor allow autonomy in discovery, or will the student be directed? Will the student be allowed to reach unique conclusions or be guided towards a particular solution to a problem? Probably more daring for the clinical area is the question of whether discovery will be accidental or planned and certainly it is very tempting to imagine (quite wrongly) the implications of employing errorful learning in patient care. It now seems appropriate that the best way of answering these questions is to give an example of how it may be implemented.

One example which is familiar to all individuals that have participated in the preceptorship of learners is that of how their teaching styles and approaches have developed over a period of time, and that with the best of intentions, no-one can ever cater for all the eventualities when teaching someone else to teach. It is in fact a discovery exercise on the part of the new teacher, and sometimes a very painful one! The development of an effective session may take the form shown in Table 5.1.

It can be seen, and indeed most of us have experienced, that the concept of timing for instance, can only be achieved through discovery and different facets of the concept will be visited as the preceptor gains more experience, so that eventually, factors other than just the session content will be taken into consideration. To return to our earlier point, we still have to take into account how we will form the concepts that we do. The example given above may be developed autonomously but more usually as the result of the direction given to us by

**Table 5.1.**   Discovery learning session development

| Activity | Developing concepts |
|---|---|
| Discovery through session planning | Theoretical content based curriculum/clinical needs<br>Approximate timing based on content<br>Teaching method appropriate to students, content and environment<br>Perceived levels of student understanding<br>Appropriateness of visual aid to content and environment |
| Discovery through session delivery | Actual levels of student understanding<br>Actual timing based on student understanding and content<br>Effectiveness of visual aids to content, environment and group<br>Effectiveness of teaching method to group, content, environment and timing |

student evaluations or through a teaching assessment. Whether we will develop our concepts in this instance in a process- or product-based manner will largely depend on what is being taught and the influences of others around us as to what outcomes need to be achieved, but it is certainly arguable that developing a teaching style is always a process activity.

## Reception learning (assimilation theory)

In this theory, Ausubel (1978) discusses four dimensions of learning:

1. Rote.
2. Reception (existing relevant cognitive structure).
3. Discovery (new information).
4. Meaningful (new and old material incorporated to form a more detailed cognitive structure).

With this theory Ausubel attempts to resolve problems facing Bruner's discovery learning, namely subject matter organisation. Ausubel presents two main principles necessary for subject matter organisation:

1. *Progressive differentiation*. General ideas are presented first (advanced organisers) followed by gradual increase in details and specificity.
2. *Integrative reconciliation*. New ideas must be consciously related to previously learned material (subsumers).

By "advanced organiser" is meant that introductory material is presented ahead of the learning task and at a higher level of abstraction and inclusiveness than the learning task itself.

Three conditions are necessary for the attainment of meaningful learning which is essential for problem solving:

1. The learner must adopt a "set" to learn the task in a meaningful manner.
2. The task must have logical meaning.
3. The learner's cognitive structures must contain specifically relevant ideas with which new material can interact.

Discovery teaching alone does not necessarily guarantee meaningful learning.

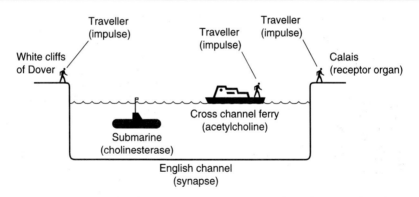

**Figure 5.2.** Example of reception learning: conduction of a nerve impulse.

Reception learning, on the other hand, is a highly functional conceptual framework for students.

*Subsumers*, which are such an essential part of the theory, enable us to integrate existing concepts with newly acquired ones. This in itself appears fairly straightforward, however, Ausubel goes on to postulate as to the existence of something that he terms "Obliterative Subsumption". In this he maintains that although much material has been forgotten residual concepts nevertheless remain and hence can be built upon. The inference of this theory as Ausubel himself points out, is that the student is the central focus of the learning process, in as much as the material to be learnt must be related to what the student already knows and that once this is established, learning will progress at a faster and more reliable rate. The implication of this is naturally that the person who is providing the instruction or experience to the student must know their student's past experiences and an honest relationship must be built up between them in order for learning to be effective. Consequently, teaching students in large groups is seen to have many drawbacks.

Ausubel accepts that not all meaningful learning involves new instances or modifications of previous learned concepts but may bear a "superalternate" relationship to a previous acquired concept. For example, superalternate learning occurs when we learn that man, cats and dogs are all mammals. As superalternate learning occurs so does integrative reconciliation, as existing concepts are rearranged into new order higher concept meanings. For example, the student recognises that different labels describe the same concept, e.g. sensory nerve/afferent nerve. A further example is given in Figure 5.2.

In this way we are enabling the student to progress in a logical manner from the known to the unknown. In other words it could be said that the student is progressing from the "concrete" to the "abstract".

# Conclusions

The introduction to this chapter pointed out that there are a variety of theories of learning and that these theories are diverse and at times totally rejecting of other theories. For instance, the humanistic school is in direct contrast to the behaviourist approach. The caution appears to be that to adopt any one method to the complete exclusion of all others could lead to vital teaching strategies being overlooked. It would appear logical to suggest that information processing, which is essentially the topic of this chapter, would be dependent upon the subject being taught, the environment in which it is being taught, time available, resources and perhaps most important of all, the personalities and preferences of both the students and preceptors. Kolb's theory, alone amongst all the others, goes to great lengths to advise us that certain learning styles are compatible with certain individuals and that care needs to be taken in how these are matched to the learning experiences available.

# Summary

Rogers uses as the basis of his theory the fact that we all have a need for positive regard, in other words, we all need to feel good about ourselves. Feeling positive regard as a result of what other people want or expect us to do results in what Rogers terms conditional positive regard.

Conditions of worth may take the form of professional behaviour, academic standards, achieving learning outcomes and even holding certain attitudes and values.

Because positive self-regard is self-esteem achieved through fulfilling the conditions placed on us by others, Rogers sees this as potentially damaging. In order to achieve true self-actualisation, Rogers advocates helping the individual to achieve unconditional self-regard.

Experiential learning theory can be described as a cyclical learning process in which Kolb describes four types of learning competencies:

1. Feeling (concrete experience competencies).
2. Perceiving (reflective observation competencies).
3. Thinking (abstract conceptualisation competencies).
4. Behaving (active experimentation competencies).

Dissatisfaction will occur if the learning style imposed on the individual is incompatible with the competency that they favour.

It should be remembered that although Kolb's theory gives us considerable insight into the differing learning styles of the individuals, it can only be used effectively if the individuals involved have been appropriately tested (Kolb, 1976; Kolb and Wolfe, 1981).

The reflexes that Pavlov described were of two types, unconditioned and conditioned reflexes.

It could be argued that all of learning can be explained in terms of operant conditioning as long as interpretation of positive reinforcement can be widened sufficiently to account for the diversity of situations that the learner may find themselves in.

Skinner devised a scheme known as "Programmed Learning", now extensively employed using computer-assisted learning techniques, so that each student may progress at their own pace.

Gagne's theory of learning has a strong behavioural slant, and describes the learning process in terms of a hierarchy as distinct from a cycle. Gagne's assertion is that the learning process focuses heavily on teacher-centred approaches, and great emphasis is placed on how information is presented.

Gestalt (insightful learning) relies heavily on the individual being able to arrive at solutions as a result of being given information which they will then organise into a complete picture.

Essentially, discovery learning is concerned with the development of concepts from processes which have enabled the individual to find common properties in objects or situations which will enable them to classify them into groups and to be able to apply general rules to them.

Ausubel presents two main principles necessary for subject matter organisation.

1. *Progressive differentiation.* General ideas are presented first (advanced organisers) followed by gradual increase in details and specificity.

2. *Integrative reconciliation*. New ideas must be consciously related to previously learned material (subsumers).

By "advanced organiser" is meant that introductory material is presented ahead of the learning task and at a higher level of abstraction and inclusiveness than the learning task itself.

# References

Ausubel, D. (1978) *Educational Psychology; a cognitive view*. New York: Rinehart & Winston.

Bloom, B.S. (1956) *Taxonomy of Educational Objectives*. Longman.

Bruner, J. (1960) *The Process of Education*. Cambridge, MA: Harvard University Press.

Condell, S.L and Elliott, N. (1989) Gagne's theory of instruction – its relevance to nurse education. *Nurse Education Today*, **9** 281–284.

Coulter, M.A. (1990) A review of two theories of learning and their application in the practice of nurse education. *Nurse Education Today*, **10**, 333–338.

Cronbach, L.J. (1966) The logic of experiments on discovery. In L.S. Shulman and E.R. Keisler (eds) *Learning by Discovery*. Chicago: Rand McNally.

Curzon, L.B. (1990) *Teaching in Further Education – An Outline of Principles and Practice*. 4th Edn. London: Cassell.

Gagne, R.M. (1974) Learning hierarchies. In H. Clarizo (ed.) *Contemporary Issues in Educational Psychology*. Allyn & Bacon.

Gagne, R.M. (1975) *Essentials of Learning for Instruction*. Hinsda, IL: The Dryden Press.

Gagne, R.M. (1985) *The Conditions of Learning and Theory of Instruction*. London: Holt Rinehart & Winston.

Kolb, D. (1976) *The Learning Style Inventory – a Technical Manual*. Boston, MA: McBer.

Kolb, D. (1984) *Experiential Learning: Experience as a Source of Learning and Development*. Englewood Cliffs, NJ: Prentice Hall.

Kolb, D. and Wolfe, D.M. (1981) Professional education and career development: a cross sectional study of adaptive competencies in experiential learning. Lifelong Learning and Adult Development Project, Final Report, Case, Weston Reserve University Cleveland, Ohio. (Cited by Laschinger 1990.)

Laschinger, H.K. (1990) Review of experiential learning theory research in the nursing profession. *Journal of Advanced Nursing*, **15**, 985–993.

Rogers, C. (1969) Freedom to Learn. Ohio, IL: Merrill.

Roger, Logan and Tierney (1981). *The Elements of Nursing*. London: Churchill Livingstone.

Skinner, B.F. (1938) *The behaviour of organisms*. New York, Appleton Century Crofts.

# chapter six

# Organising material

## Introduction

For the the purposes of the discussion here, two major factors that have an effect on organising material will be dealt with, namely memory and perception. Both of these factors are crucial to the planning process involved for any session, and ignoring them can lead to poorly conducted and ineffective sessions where the participants have not been able to meet their learning outcomes.

Other factors such as attitudes, motivation and communication have been covered elsewhere in the text, and these are equally important to the discussion.

## Memory

One of the most obvious components which affects learning must be the ability to remember information and experiences. The process of memory is, as with many other areas in psychology, still the subject of ongoing research, and although numerous theories have been expounded on the subject, only two major theories will be explored here, namely the *multi-store model* and the *working memory model*. The memory process is only part of the equation in terms of learning in as much as the individual will need to be able to utilise information which has been stored, in a meaningful way.

It has been the subject of much debate that the ability to remember and the ability to learn are two distinct entities, particularly if we refer to Gagne's Hierarchy of Learning which identifies the most sophisticated form of learning as problem solving. To return to discussions in earlier chapters, problem solving must involve the utilisation of memory but it is rather the ability to be able to integrate new knowledge in order to solve problems in novel situations that could be said to epitomise learning in its truer sense. A nurse, for instance, who has managed to remember significant amounts of physiology and is completely unable to translate this into effective patient care has not been able to carry out such an integration. Our discussion will by necessity begin with some basic principles of memory which will have an impact firstly on how the sessions are prepared for the student, and secondly how the student will deal with this information. It must be stressed that this subject cannot be read in isolation from other factors affecting learning.

Our starting point both in terms of aiding our understanding of the subject and also presenting the reader with a more complete picture of memory, is its physiological basis.

## The physiological basis of memory

The search for a physiological explanation of memory is by no means a new venture, and indeed the phenomenon of memory loss associated with head injury and various neurological disorders is familiar to most of us. Various structures do appear to play a major part in the memory process, although the picture is, at present incomplete.

The hippocampus, which is situated in the forebrain has been linked with memory and learning, and along with the neurotransmitter, glutamate, is seen as an important centre for learning (Gustaffson and Wigstrom, 1988), although it seems much more likely that it is only part of the system. Thompson (1978) has suggested that the frontal cortex, the posterior thalamus, and the amygdala are all responsible for fear-initiated responses, whilst the occipital cortex, hippocampus and mammilary bodies are important for cognitive mapping. The basal ganglia are responsible for sensorimotor integration, and the cerebellum, parietal cortex and the anterior thalamus are concerned with somatosensory function.

From a functional viewpoint, it has been suggested that learning involves the formation of new circuits within the brain (Ungar, 1974), and others have suggested that changes in RNA could be the key to the physiological basis of learning. The true picture is immensely complicated, and at times, the evidence points us in several different directions, although it is highly likely that, given time, a complex interrelated system will be discovered.

# Memory and learning

## Short-term and long-term memory

It is a common characteristic of theories of memory (e.g. Broadbent, 1958; Atkinson and Shiffrin, 1968) that two distinct types of memory exist, namely short- and long-term memory. Quite how they are organised and the fine detail of how they function are the features distinguishing between the theories. In its most basic form (Miller, 1956), short-term memory is said to have a small capacity (five to nine pieces of information) which can be retained for only a short period of time (approximately 30 seconds). This is in contrast to the long-term memory where items may be stored throughout the individual's life span.

## Encoding in short-term and long-term memory

What appears to dominate in the short-term memory is the *acoustic code*. Conrad (1964) noted that there were significant characteristics about the errors that subjects made when recalling letters from the short-term memory, in as much as they tended to substitute letters which sounded similar to those letters which were actually presented (M for N and B for T). This phenomenon even occurred if the letters were presented visually rather than verbally, implying that the letters were held in the short-term memory in terms of their acoustic rather than visual properties. The acoustic coding dominance in short-term memory appears to be further supported when words are presented (Baddeley, 1966b) where the results reflected an acoustic rather than a visual or semantic coding system.

In the equivalent long-term memory study (Baddeley, 1966a) it was found that semantically similar words were remembered poorly, suggesting that in long-term memory words were remembered in terms of their meanings, leading to the conclusion that semantic similarity affects the long-term memory (Baddeley and Dale, 1966). Therefore the long-term memory has a preferred semantic code and the short-term memory has a preferred acoustic code, but other codes may be used, although to a much lesser extent.

## Storage and attention

The manner in which information is stored is a matter of some controversy, and is in many ways linked to how we attend to information. Two models will be discussed here.

Possibly the better known of the two models is that proposed by Atkinson and Shiffrin (1968), which describes a multi-store comprising sensory registers, a short-term store (STS) and a long-term store (LTS) (Figure 6.1). Information is initially received and stored for as little as a fraction of a second in the *sensory memory* or register. From here, information may either be lost, or attended to and transferred to an STS. Once again the information may be lost after about 20–30 seconds, this time by a process of displacement. There is a way, however, to prevent its loss from the STS, and this is by "rehearsal", which will increase the possibility of transfer to the LTS. Once in the LTS, information may be stored permanently, and may be retrieved when needed. Alternatively, the information may decay or may become confused with other similar memory traces.

## Working memory model

An alternative to the "multi-store" model described by Atkinson and Shiffrin has been proposed; the "working memory" model proposes four separate components to replace the STS (Figure 6.2).

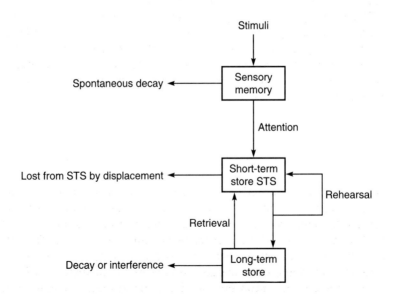

**Figure 6.1.** Information storage ("multi-store") model (adapted from Atkinson and Shiffrin, 1968).

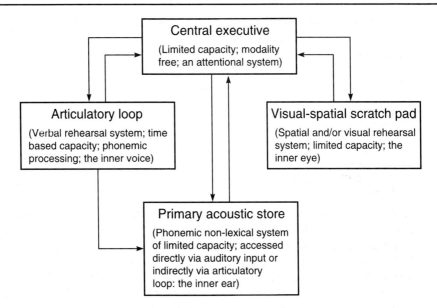

**Figure 6.2.** "Working memory" model (from Cohen *et al.*, 1988).

The *central executive* has, to a large extent, control over the other components, although the primary acoustic store is to an extent dependent upon certain actions of the articulatory loop. The central executive can store information for short periods of time, can process information from sensory inputs in a variety of ways and is involved in tasks such as reading, writing, problem solving, mental arithmetic and learning. In other words, the central executive is involved whenever attention is demanded.

The *articulatory loop* not only holds the words we are about to say, but also acts as a rehearsal loop similar to that in the Atkinson–Shiffrin model, and is used whenever we verbally repeat material in order to memorise it. It therefore deals with the articulation of verbal material and is considered as an "inner voice".

The *visual–spatial scratch pad* is responsible for dealing with visual and spatial information. It has a limited capacity, and utilises rehearsal. It can be regarded as the "inner eye".

The *primary acoustic store* is dependent upon the articulatory loop for the translation of visual information in an acoustic code, but deals with auditory information directly. This store can be used when reading and the printed matter can be "heard" as we read. This store can be referred to as the "inner ear".

# Retrieval

The retrieval of information and the nature of forgetting can be considered together for the purposes of this discussion. Retrieval from the short-term memory is a very fast process, not "instant", being dependent upon the number of items stored there. In other words, a search needs to be carried out (Sternberg, 1966). Information is lost from the short-term memory by a process of displacement when the storage capacity is exceeded.

As far as the long-term memory is concerned, analogies can be made which may serve to explain some of the processes involved. For instance, imagine a large room full of filing cabinets which in their turn are full of files, and further imagine that we are asked to locate a particular file. Our chances of finding the file will become considerably more remote if there are no labels on the filing cabinets to indicate their contents, and if the files themselves have been placed in the cabinets in a random fashion, our failure will become almost inevitable. The same sort of outcome can be expected when using a word processor when someone has just labelled the files as "1", "2", "3", etc., with no clue as to their contents. Accurate naming of files in both instances will increase our chances of finding the file, and also if the contents are arranged in a logical manner (e.g. if the file is labelled "mortgage" we might expect to find not only the contract from the bank, but also the surveyor's report, legal documents and details such as mortgage account statements).

Similarly, retrieval from the long-term memory can be said to be, at least in part, dependent on how it was organised in the first place (Bower *et al.*, 1969). Categorising the material that we encode has been found to aid recall, and this is seen perhaps most clearly when attempting to learn material, such as that relating to intestinal obstruction, which will encompass many different conditions.

This organisation of material has also been investigated by Tulving (1968), who suggested that we may group information in terms of their relationships (*primary organisation*), and that we may further remember information by categorical or associative means (*secondary organisation*). The categorical organisation has already been mentioned, but the associative aspect is concerned with the associations that we may form between different pieces of information, such as opposites. In considering the organisation of material, it can be deduced that the responsibilities of teaching both patients and junior staff lie not only in the accuracy of information, but also in the manner and order in which it is presented.

The manner in which we encode can also have a bearing on how information is forgotten. A poorly delivered lecture which does not attempt to make links with the recipients' past experience is less likely to be remembered. The information should be made relevant to the individual, because there is a tendency for the memory trace to decay over time as new information causes interference, unless the previously learned material is being used either in a practical sense, or as a foundation for further learning. A good example of this is when we are taught a subject such as psychology or physiology in complete isolation from our main area of study: before much time has elapsed, the learning of our more specialist subject has caused interference with previously learned material. This could have been avoided if sufficient account had been taken of the relationships between each subject when it was taught.

The question still remains as to how the information is brought into our conscious thought. The process involved appears to revolve around the presentation of cues which were present at the time of learning. These are most commonly words or phrases, and could be likened to looking for and finding a file in our filing cabinet with a title, and then finding the information that we require inside.

Many of us, when referring to material learned many years previously, have expressed the sentiment that "it soon comes back", particularly when referring to a "work" situation, and in this instance, a return to the contextual surroundings (such as a hospital ward) may act as a cue. In other words, if we return to the area where certain information was encoded then we are more likely to remember it (Estes, 1972).

Wiseman and Tulving (1976) have further developed this type of theory by suggesting that the relationship between storage and retrieval can be likened to a lock and key, with the lock representing the information stored in the memory trace, and the key representing the information available at the time of retrieval. This theory emphasises the need for there to be a match between the stored information and the retrieval information by the "to be remembered" item being encoded

"... with respect to the context in which it is studied, producing a unique trace which incorporates information from both target and context. For the 'to be remembered' item to be retrieved, the cue information must appropriately match the trace of the item in context".

This "encoding specificity principle" implies that during learning there should be a degree of matching to the anticipated retrieval code. For example, teaching a patient to use a syringe merely by showing them drawings of the syringe is likely to lead to some confusion because the encoded information from the drawings is likely to be an inappropriate retrieval cue.

## Emotional factors in forgetting

The manner in which emotion makes us forget information can in part be explained by the encoding specificity principle discussed earlier, with information being remembered if the subject is in a similar mood to when the information was originally encoded, although this is by no means the only possible explanation.

The psychoanalytic explanation for forgetting could, in some instances be that the experience was so unpleasant that the individual represses it in order to protect themselves, and this form of defence mechanism is particularly prevalent in childhood.

Possibly the most obvious explanation would be that retrieval is made difficult because a strong emotion (not necessarily a bad one) is causing interference with the retrieval mechanism.

Much, if not all, of the behaviour that we exhibit as adults has been shaped in earlier life, and learning is no exception. The experiences that we have all had during our school years, for instance, will inevitably leave their mark either in a positive or negative way, and equally, some experiences may leave us with fairly neutral feelings about a subject, how it was taught and how we feel about learning it. There is the possibility though that unpleasant learning experiences, far from making us unable to retrieve the information later, will prevent it being stored in the first place.

## Implications for planning a teaching session

1. Plan the speed of the presentation – introduce new information slowly.
2. Do not try to cram information into the session.
3. Try to work to time, particularly when approaching meal breaks!
4. Try not to teach for more than about 20 minutes without changing activities (introduce group work, discussion, etc.).
5. Utilise students' knowledge and experience – it will make storing information easier.
6. Reinforce information visually (e.g. overhead projector, handouts, or even with their permission, patients/clients).
7. Give a clear summary as the information covered at the end of the session is most likely to be remembered.
8. Remember that the material may be entirely new to the student, so give time for questions and for them to integrate the information.

Much of the work carried out on memory appears, as seen, to point us in the same direction in so far as the organisation of material seems to play a crucial role in helping us to encode, store and retrieve information. Put another way, the way the individual perceives information in the first place has a bearing on whether they will remember it in the future. Our discussion will therefore be directed towards the organisation of material, and in doing so, the Gestalt approach to learning will be briefly examined.

# Perception and Gestalt psychology

Gestalt, or "insightful learning", is concerned with the relationship between subject matter organisation and its effect on learning. In its most fundamental sense, Gestalt (meaning "form") psychology is concerned with the formation of patterns and how individuals perceive them. For the purposes of this discussion, the "Law of Pragnanz", a corner-stone of Gestalt psychology, will be examined.

## The Law of Pragnanz

Gestalt psychologists, such as Koffka (1935), have placed considerable importance on "perception in terms of organisational and configurational properties" (Dember and Warm, 1979). The Law of Pragnanz, briefly, is the basic principle that suggests that the perceptual response in any given situation will be the most economical one possible (Hochberg, 1971), and that these responses depend on certain grouping principles.

Pictorially, these grouping principles are given below, and are readily identifiable. Just as individuals respond to such grouping with pictorial information, so the same rules apply to material that they are attempting to learn:

1. Symmetry.
2. Similarity.
3. Proximity.
4. Closure.

### Symmetry

The most obvious characteristic that material should have in order that it is interpreted effectively is symmetry. We are more likely to dissect out symmetrical rather than asymmetrical patterns. This is expressed pictorially, in Figure 6.3, with the symmetrical patterns being noticed in preference to the asymmetrical ones.

Learning material should therefore be organised in a symmetrical manner, enabling the student to be able to perceive it as a complete entity. In its simplest form, a teaching session,

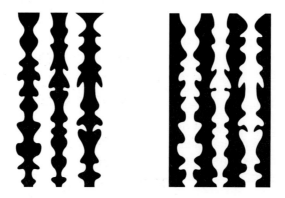

**Figure 6.3.** Symmetry. (Left, black patterns are symmetrical. Right, white patterns are asymmetrical.)

for instance, should have a clearly distinguishable and sequential introduction, development and summary.

## Similarity

The elements of any collection of visual or learning materials will be grouped in terms of similar properties as perceived by the individual. Pictorially, the Figure 6.4 will normally be interpreted as three separate, equally sized squares rather than as five different sized squares/rectangles.

As far as learning material is concerned, perceived similarities will tend to be grouped together. This can be facilitated, and hence make material easier to learn through effective session planning, but perhaps more importantly, through curriculum planning. Difficulties in learning may emerge due to semantic similarities such as aphagia and aphasia, haematemasis and haemoptesis, etc. Learning the semantic origins of such words may help to reduce the confusion.

## Proximity

We tend to form groups of information that are spatially close together. Pictorially, we may look at Figure 6.5 and conclude that the wider gaps constitute spaces, whereas the narrower gaps constitute "columns".

With learning material, this principle can be used when planning a programme of experience so that information that is presented within a module will be learnt as a complete entity, rather than having it randomly scattered throughout the experience, in which case, associations may not be made and gaps in learning may result.

## Closure

The tendency that we have to perceive figures as complete and symmetrical even though they may be incomplete is again equally as applicable to learning material as it is to visually presented material. This is shown pictorially in Figure 6.6.

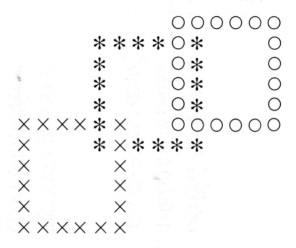

**Figure 6.4.** Similarity.

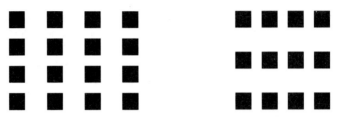

**Figure 6.5.** Proximity.

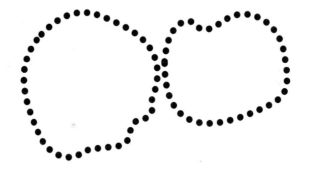

**Figure 6.6.** Closure.

## Conclusions

The ways in which the individual organises material is of crucial importance in learning. It appears that the teaching session should take account not only of the rate at which information is given, but must also recognise the fact that past experience and external factors can affect how information is dealt with, if at all.

The planning of a session is therefore not as centred on the academic information as would first appear, but is equally geared to how the information is presented and over what time span. The need of most people trying to teach their subject, at least initially, is to ensure that they have covered the information in sufficient depth, and this will frequently lead to information overload.

Quite apart from the memory aspects of learning, the expert will often depart from the laws of perception that should govern teaching as they jump backwards and forwards in an attempt to explain concepts that they thought their students were conversant with.

## Summary

One of the most obvious components which affects learning must be the ability to remember information and experiences.

The ability to be able to integrate new knowledge in order to solve problems in novel situations that could be said to epitomise learning in its truer sense.

It is a common characteristic of theories of memory (e.g. Broadbent, 1958; Atkinson and Shiffrin, 1968) that two distinct types of memory exist, namely short- and long-term memory.

Atkinson and Shiffrin (1968), describe a multi-store comprising sensory registers, a short-term store and a long-term store.

An alternative to the "multi-store" model described by Atkinson and Shiffrin has been proposed; the "working memory" model proposes four separate components to replace the short-term store.

Retrieval from the short-term memory is a very fast process, but not "instant", being dependent upon the number of items stored there.

Retrieval from the long-term memory can be said to be, at least in part, dependent on how it was organised in the first place.

Tulving (1968) suggested that we may group information in terms of their relationships (primary organisation), and that we may further remember information by categorical or associative means (secondary organisation).

Gestalt, or "insightful learning", is concerned with the relationship between subject matter organisation and its effect on learning.

The Law of Pragnanz, briefly, is the basic principle that suggests that the perceptual response in any given situation will be the most economical one possible (Hochberg, 1971), and that these responses depend on certain grouping principles.

# Related activity

Observe a teaching session given by a colleague, and make short notes on the following:

1. Was there a definite introduction that attempted to put the session into context?
2. Was the students' previous experience and knowledge taken into account, and if so, how was this done?
3. How was symmetry demonstrated?
4. Did activities change throughout the session, and if so, what time intervals were involved, and what were the activities?
5. Were any learning checks made by the facilitator of the session, and if so, what were they (e.g. questions, practice)?
6. Were there any aspects of the session that the students were required to complete or practice, if so, what?
7. Did the session follow a logical sequence?
8. Did the session have a coherent conclusion?

# References

An asterix indicates a standard text or article.

*Atkinson, R.C and Shiffrin, R.M (1968) Human memory: a proposed system and its control processes. In K.W. Spence and J.T. Spence (eds), *The Psychology of Learning and Motivation*, Vol. 2, Academic Press.

*Baddeley, A.D. (1966a) The influence of acoustic and semantic similarity on long term memory for word sequences. *Quarterly Journal of Experimental Psychology*, **18**, 362–365.

*Baddeley, A.D (1966b) Short term memory for word sequences as a function of acoustic, semantic and formal similarity. *Quarterly Journal of Experimental Psychology*, **20**, 249–264.

*Baddeley, A.D. and Dale, H.C.A. (1966) The effect of semantic similarity on retroactive interference in long and short term memory. *Journal of Verbal Learning and Verbal Behaviour*, **5**, 417–420.

Bower, G.H., Clark, M.C., Winzenz, D. and Lesgold, D. (1969) Hierarchical retrieval schemes in recall of categorised word lists. *Journal of Verbal Learning and Verbal Behaviour*, **8**, 323–343.

Broadbent (1958) *Perception and Communication*. Oxford: Pergamon.

Cohen, G., Eysenck, M.W. and LeVoi, M.E. (1986) *Memory – a Cognitive Approach*. Open University Press.

Conrad, R. (1964) Acoustic confusion in immediate memory. *British Journal of Psychology*, **55**, 75–84.

Dember, W.N. and Warm, J.S. (1979) Psychology of Perception, 2nd edn. Ohio, IL: Holt, Rinehart and Winston.

Estes, W.K. (1972) An associative basis for coding and organisation in memory. In A.W. Meltron and E. Martin (eds) *Coding Processes in Human Memory*. Washington DC: Winston.

Gustaffson, B. and Wigstrom, H. (1988) Physiological mechanisms underlying long term potentiation. *Trends in Neuroscience*, **11**, 156–162.

Hochberg, J.E. (1971) Perception: I. color and shape. In J.W. Kling & L.A. Riggs (eds.) *Woodworth and Schlosberg's Experimental Psychology*. **3rd edn**. New York: Holt, Rinehart and Winston.

Koffka, K. (1935) *Principles of Gestalt Psychology*. New York: Harcourt.

Miller, G.A. (1956) The magical number seven plus or minus two: some limits on our capacity for processing information. *Psychological Review*, **63**, 81–97.

Sternberg, S. (1966) High speed scanning in human memory. *Science*. **153**, 652–654.

Thompson (1978) Localisation of a passive avoidance memory system in the white rat. *Physiological Psychology*, **4**, 311–324.

Tulving, E. (1968) Theoretical issues in free recall. In T. Dixon and D. Horton (eds). *Verbal Behaviour and General Behaviour Theory*. Englewood Cliffs, NJ: Prentice Hall.

Ungar (1974) Molecular coding of memory. *Life Sciences*, **14**, 595–604.

Wiseman, S. and Tulving E. (1976) Encoding specificity: relation between recall superiority and recognition failure. *Journal of Experimental Psychology: Human Learning; Memory*, **2**, 349–361.

# chapter seven

# Planning a learning experience

## Introduction

It could be argued that most teaching in the clinical area deals with skills, including interpersonal and management skills. It is necessary to recognise skills not just as an entity which encompasses the physical elements of an activity but in its widest sense, encompassing even more traditionally humanist aspects such as counselling, interviewing and dealing with relatives. This does not of course exclude the fact that some theoretical teaching/learning may take place in order to supplement and enhance the skills.

The discussion on perception highlighted the fact that in order for us to learn, some structure must be inherent in the material being presented. Even with the most humanistic approaches, there should be an identified starting point, development and definable end point in order to give the session structure. Usually, and for the purposes of this text, this is identified as introduction, development and conclusions.

The whole concept that any session where there is to be a structured mentor–learner interaction requires planning is relatively straightforward. The factors which affect learning included in Chapters two and six, as well as the theories of learning (Chapter five), complicate what appears to be a simple concept into one in which the needs of the students, the subject matter, the environment and indeed the needs and preferences of the mentor/preceptor will all have an effect. It is not always the case that teaching strategies are ideally matched with learners' needs (Dux, 1989; Burnard and Morrison, 1991), and factors such as role modelling and past experiences will have a bearing on how information is to be imparted.

Theories of learning, particularly when considering the humanistic and behaviourist approaches, will quite naturally have far-reaching implications for the method of teaching used. Additionally, it seems likely that the personality of the preceptor will be a major contributing factor in the choice of method and consequently its likelihood of success. A word of caution is appropriate at this juncture, even if it states the obvious, namely, not everyone is good at using every method and an inability to be effective using one approach should not be regarded as a sign of failure on the part of the preceptor.

This chapter uses as its basis the underlying principle that the vast number of teaching strategies require a similar planning stage and that these can be applied to both formal and informal approaches. The way in which different methods are presented is perhaps unavoidably misleading in so far as it is easy to assume that prescriptive approaches are being advocated. This is most certainly not the case as it is relatively rare for most experienced preceptors to use any method in its textbook form, but rather to bring their own past experiences, preferences and personality into their teaching style.

# Factors to consider prior to planning your session

1. Which method of presentation best suits the subject?
2. How long do you have for your presentation?
3. How many participants will there be?
4. The environment.
5. Time of day.
6. Previous knowledge/experience of the subject within the group.
7. Enthusiasm/motivation of the group for the subject to be covered.
8. Resources available.

Naturally, depending on the the above factors, the teacher will have to decide what their role is going to be during the session. It is too simple just to say that teaching will take place. It is perhaps more appropriate to describe the process as a facilitation of learning, and as such, the role of the teacher can be considered in much broader terms.

One way of looking at the role of the teacher and the strategies that may be used is to consider the type of learning that will occur, and this in turn is usually dependent on the subject matter and students (Steinaker and Bell, 1979). In this experiential learning theory, Steinaker and Bell organise learning into the following taxonomy:

1. Exposure.
2. Participation.
3. Identification.
4. Internalisation.
5. Dissemination.

# Exposure

This initial part of the learning process is concerned with developing a consciousness of the experience. This is something that we are all aware of when confronted with new situations and subjects. This exposure can take the form of seeing a procedure done for the first time, being shown a piece of equipment, or even in some circumstances, listening to a formal talk or being involved in a discussion.

In this "exposure" phase, the role of the teacher should be to facilitate effective observation, and even to set the scene for the student to begin to explore. The teaching methods used here may range from a formal lecture to a tour of the department.

# Participation

During this part of the process the student explores and they become more involved in the experience as a result. It does not imply competence, but the teacher's role is that of a catalyst so that competence is aimed for.

The role of the teacher in this case will be that of an agent who facilitates recall, helps the student to expand their knowledge base, and of course, facilitates participation. In practice-based learning, the teacher must be able to give effective feedback as well as (at times) the more formal modes of teaching in order to build on what has been learnt.

# Identification

Active participation typifies this stage. The learner develops competence and as further practice follows, so the subject matter is reinforced.

The teacher's role at this stage is that of moderator as the student utilises concepts and observes the results of their actions and learning. Through structured discussion and informal interactions, further ramifications can be explored.

# Internalisation

Internalisation occurs when the experience becomes part of the individual's "repartee" and influences aspects of their life. What was once a novel and strange experience is now part of everyday work, and continues to influence it.

The role of the teacher at this stage is that of sustainer and should be helping the student not only to consolidate their knowledge but also to help them extend their skills to more novel situations. As such, teaching strategies should be aimed at facilitating debate, discussion and even the exploration and utilisation of knowledge and skills in a safe environment, through games, simulations and role play.

# Dissemination

At this stage, the student is passing their knowledge onto others. In attempting to influence other people the education process enters a crucial stage in as far as bad or incorrect knowledge as well as accurate and complete knowledge may be passed on.

The role of the teacher during this dissemination stage is that of critic. The dissemination of information to others will probably involve the students themselves in a teaching role, sometimes formally, but often others will learn from them by observation.

# Choosing the teaching strategy

The factors that should be taken into account when planning a session will centre around several key areas. The first area, namely the role that the teacher will play, has been discussed earlier, and will naturally be dependent on what is being attempted in terms of learning outcomes.

The preferences of the teacher for one strategy over another need to be considered in the light of the reasons why they are being preferred rather than what is being preferred. Some authors (e.g. Dux, 1989) have urged teachers to examine their motives in choosing a particular method, whilst others (e.g Burnard and Morrison, 1991) have suggested a mismatch between teacher- and student-preferred strategies. With this in mind, it must also be accepted that we can all use certain strategies better than others.

The level of the material presented is quite naturally an important factor, but perhaps more important are the abilities of the students to cope with the information. It is tempting to assume that all students at a certain stage in the course will be able to solve problems, or at least will be able to exercise reasoning abilities when entering the course. This is a somewhat precarious presumption to make, as it has been suggested (e.g. Klaassens, 1992; Frisch, 1987) that as many as 50% to 80% may be functioning at a lower level at least during the initial part of training. Care therefore needs to be taken not to overburden the new student with problem-solving exercises at the beginning, but rather to reserve them for a time when a more accurate assessment of the student's abilities can be made.

The content of the session will often lend itself to a specific method although again this cannot be looked at in isolation from other factors. Teaching cardiopulmonary resuscitation (CPR) to students who have never seen it before may lend itself to a structured lecture and demonstration. Periodic updates of CPR skills, although covering substantially the same material, may utilise a "game" format to achieve its outcomes.

Finally, a word needs to be said about the preceptor–student relationship. If there is a high degree of trust involved in the relationship, this may guide the preceptor towards more humanistic approaches for certain subjects, e.g. bereavement, where the student's own experiences may form the basis of the session. In cases where the relationship is either new or has difficulties, then this may present problems and restrictions when choosing the strategy. If this is the case, then the relationship difficulties should be resolved before the programme of learning is commenced. This may mean changing the preceptor.

# Teaching strategies

## The lecture

The lecture, despite being teacher centred, is one of the more popular methods favoured by both students and teachers (Dux, 1989). It does indeed have some important contributions to make to learning in the clinical setting as well as some major drawbacks. Certainly used on its own in an unadapted form, it is typically a good example of a pedagogical, didactic, restricted feedback method. On the positive side, this method does allow for large amounts of information to be conveyed in a short period of time and it is the preferred strategy for some students, probably because of the security it offers by virtue of the lack of self-disclosure required on their part.

It is difficult in some instances to avoid using some form of formal lecture and this may usually be a short exposition to introduce the subject. In the clinical setting, this most usefully should be followed by learning occurring by other methods (e.g. experientially). Curzon (1990) suggests that a formal lecture may be used to explain a problem and its possible solutions or to present a thesis, although in its wider context, it may be an integral part of more student-centred sessions. This is particularly the case when the students have little or no knowledge to apply to a given situation and as such frequently forms the basis of demonstrations.

Although a period of questions and answers should be included at the end of a formal lecture, if this is the sole method of teaching, a more advisable strategy is to use the informal lecture method where student–preceptor interaction is encouraged throughout. This is obviously far more preferable as it allows difficulties to be overcome as they are encountered rather than running the risk of the student losing track of the session halfway through.

# Seminar

The seminar is, typically, a combination of formal exposition and discussion and can be used for sessions where a series of papers is to be presented, different aspects of care are to be covered or even where students have reviewed the literature on a subject and wish to present it in a structured way. There are of course many other applications, many of which would be redundant in the clinical area, mainly because of time constraints, but all can follow the same basic format. An example of a seminar format on the subject of caring for a patient with multiple sclerosis could be:

1. Introduction to the whole session

2. Introduction to disordered physiology
3. Development of above theme
4. Conclusions
5. Discussion
6. Summing-up by group leader

7. Introduction to medical care
8. Development of above theme
9. Conclusions
10. Discussion
11. Summing-up by group leader

12. Introduction to nursing care
13. Development of above theme
14. Conclusions
15. Discussion
16. Summing-up by group leader

17. Introduction to the patient's perspective
18. Development of above theme
19. Conclusions
20. Discussion
21. Summing-up by group leader

22. Conclusions from group/group leader

Although it may look rather long-winded and cumbersome, it should be remembered that the presentations may be only very short if so desired, but may be given by either different members of the group or by experts. The seminar can be a good way for groups to share the results of their research into a topic, and particularly if some form of handout can be arranged for each presentation, may actually lead to the easing of tension created by the strain on individuals having to research major topics in isolation.

# Demonstration

On first inspection, the demonstration of a skill would appear to be, at least in the initial part of the session, rather teacher centred. It is most certainly true that the demonstration involves, by its very nature, a "visual explanation of facts, concepts and procedures" (Quinn, 1988), and that by the end of the session, the student should have some idea about the proper way to, for instance give an injection. Four points need to be made here in order to put this method into context.

Firstly, the demonstration method has the same basic "introduction, development and conclusion" format that other methods have. Secondly, discovery learning can be an effective device to employ and this can be used to good effect when asking students to apply concepts that they may already have learned to the situation in hand. Many demonstrations can be carried out in the safe environment of a treatment room, where mistakes made by the student in the initial part of the session can form the basis of the rest of the session and certainly help to put the session into context.

Thirdly, some skills, for instance communicating with patients, will be modified by the students in accordance with their own personalities and attitudes, and the learning process will be more protracted and complicated as a result. Consequently, the student, even though they have been taught the basic skill of admitting a patient near the beginning of a module, may only achieve complete competence a few modules later as their experience grows and their own style has emerged.

Finally, it would appear that a demonstration of a skill needs, in order to be effective, to include interaction between the preceptor and the student, and as such sessions which rely solely on the use of video, etc., may not be as effective (Baldwin *et al.*, 1991).

## Discussion

On the face of it the discussion appears to be the easiest of all the teaching strategies to set up and run, and it has to be said, that with adequate planning, its execution should be relatively straightforward. A discussion format can be used effectively to help students to understand concepts that may have been covered in a previous session, as a debriefing exercise to other strategies, or just to explore facets of a topic, particularly where personal experiences and attitudes may help others to learn.

Discussion can also be used to help students to explore ethical issues such as euthanasia, and when this sort of topic is approached, then it may be beneficial to use a special sort of discussion method known as "structured controversy" (e.g. Pederson, 1992; Johnson and Johnson, 1988). With this method (see below) it is suggested that there is a positive influence on students' skills in forming a perspective, arguing logically and reaching a consensus.

Generally speaking, the discussion method may help to change attitudes, improve communication skills and to promote critical thinking. By sharing experiences and knowledge, problem-solving behaviours may also be promoted.

## Role play

Role play is used most frequently when the preceptor wants the students to be able to empathise with a particular group of people (parents in casualty, a patient being admitted, etc.). The method will consist broadly of participants taking on a particular role in a given situation, and, with the scenario and characters explained, playing out the roles.

This method can be used in a variety of sessions, but without adequate briefing beforehand, and debriefing afterwards, it will be of little use. The relationship between the preceptor and the student is crucial, as significant self-disclosures may take place under certain circumstances (for instance if the exercise is exploring subjects such as bereavement).

Role play should be used with the consensus of the group, with no-one being coerced into participating against their will.

## Games and simulations

A simulation is essentially an extended role play with structure and rules. Typically, the setting is prescribed and constraints are given to a group of people. Such simulations are common in management studies. One of the characteristics that distinguishes it from a role-play situation is that definite decisions will need to be made, and an end product is usually definable.

Games can vary from a simulation where individuals are in competition with each other, to board- and computer-based games which may have one or multiple participants. Uses for a game format have been found in teaching skills and areas as unlikely as hospital standards and policies (Felder, 1992).

## Case studies

Case studies can be used either as a teaching or assessment strategy, and facilitate problem-solving. For a more detailed account of the uses and classifications of case studies, the reader is referred to Chapter nine.

## Group work

The term "group work" is a misleading one as it suggests a single teaching method, whereas the term encompasses several different types of activity, including buzz groups (where the group will generate ideas by "brainstorming"), project groups, discussion groups (student led) and cooperative learning groups (an interactive strategy used to foster critical thinking). These methods tend to be student centred and tend to follow approximately the same pattern of planning.

Quite apart from the motivational aspects of group work, these methods are used to improve communication, foster cooperation between students, provide peer support and of course to share ideas. In achieving this it is hoped to facilitate problem solving and critical thinking.

## Planning a teaching session

This could perhaps be more appropriately entitled "planning a learning session", as the word "teaching" tends to conjure up images of more formal teacher-centred approaches. If the taxonomy offered by Steinaker and Bell, along with the role of the teacher, is accepted then more student-centred approaches need to be encompassed.

Generally though, most sessions can be divided up into introduction, development and conclusions, which in the more didactic of formats can be translated into:

1. Tell them what you are going to tell them!
2. Tell them!
3. Tell them what you've told them!

In terms of a more student-centred approach it can be interpreted thus:

1. Negotiate content and agree outcomes.
2. Facilitate learning.
3. Review outcomes in light of the session.

In order that effective planning can take place, it is a good idea to use some form of planning format. Although, as will be seen, different methods will have varying emphasis and strategies at each stage, most individuals like to use the same planning format for all sessions.

## Reasons for using a teaching plan

1. Encourages rationalisation of notes.
2. Promotes logical thought and anticipates possible problems.
3. Encourages a logical sequence and development.
4. Helps to indicate the method that should be used.
5. Ensures that resources are ready and available when needed.

Note that the plan shown in Figure 7.1 is used as an example only and may need to be adapted by the individual.

# Aspects of planning different teaching methods

## Introduction

The introduction to a session will naturally depend on factors already mentioned, but perhaps more importantly, whether the session is student or teacher centred. For either session, an introduction of the teacher as well as any introductions within the group should be carried out.

For more teacher-centred methods, such as formal lectures and demonstrations, within the introduction the students should be informed of the length of the session, areas to be covered and what they should hope to gain from the session. Using a student-centred approach, some discussion should take place regarding the level, content and even method that the students feel would be most beneficial to them.

Although the length of the session may be determined by workload, it should be remembered that learning will continue beyond the session and it may be possible to discuss at this stage how further support and teaching may occur. Using a taxonomy approach such as that described earlier (Steinaker and Bell, 1979) may help to begin this planning process.

This part of the session can be used to develop a rapport with the group by discussing their previous knowledge and experience of the subject, concerns regarding the subject, etc.

Specifically, introductions to the following, more commonly used methods can have the characteristics identified.

## TEACHING PLAN

Subject:                                              Name:

Presentation Method:                                  Date:

Venue:                                                Time:

### Details of Participants/Audience

Date (for updating purposes)

Number of Students:

Course Title:

Previous Experience/Stage of Course

| Room Arrangement | A/V Resources: |
| --- | --- |
| | |

### Learning Outcomes:

Presentation Method/Content:

| Time | Stages | Main Points | A/V Aids | Self-Evaluation |
| --- | --- | --- | --- | --- |
| | | | | |

References

Remarks for Future Planning:

**Figure 7.1.** Teaching plan.

## Lecture

Inform students as to what information is being covered and why and in what depth. Expected learning outcomes should be given and explained. If the lecture is examining a problem along with a variety of solutions (such as the problem of nurses practising in conflicting ways, and the solutions being the use of a variety of nursing models), then the problem itself could form the basis of the introduction.

## Demonstration

When demonstrating a skill, once again, the learning outcomes must be explained. Often, these will offer little room for individuality if there are limited (or only one) set of actions leading to competence of that skill. The reasons for learning the skill should be explained along with other information such as where it can be used and even the advantages of carrying out the skill in the way they are about to learn.

## Seminar

The seminar method will often have to be explained to the students in the introduction. Often a seminar can be used to explore several aspects of a subject (for instance, *in vitro* fertilisation looked at from the biological, psychological, ethical and legal viewpoints). The students need to be aware of their role, and the importance of discussion during the seminar, as well as the reasons for presenting it in this way.

Strictly speaking, the seminar will have a series of "introductions" (as well as the other two components) with each aspect of the session, and it is perhaps more advisable to explain the learning outcomes relevant to that part of the session as it is encountered.

## Discussion

The reasons why a discussion method may be used have already been considered, and the particular reason for its use with the student group in question should be made clear. This could indeed be the basis of the learning outcomes and it may be the case that the students (if appropriate) may wish to negotiate these themselves if, for instance, this method is being used as a follow-up session to an experience or formal teaching session.

## Role play

The introduction to a role-play session usually will not include the learning outcomes, partly because it would detract from the spontaneity of the situation, but mostly because they are difficult to predict, although the reasons for its use should be explained.

The willingness of the students to participate in the exercise should be ascertained, and those not wishing to take part should be active observers of the exercise (Quinn, 1988). The rules, time constraints and format should be explained. A brief should be given to each of the participants. Time must be given for discussion before the session begins.

## Simulations/games

The introduction to games and simulations is aimed towards explaining the rules, time constraints, any equipment or documentation and other general conditions. Learning outcomes as such may be difficult to identify in the traditional sense, but nevertheless, the student should be guided towards outcomes that will demonstrate problem-solving skills and even self-evaluation. If using a game format, the student will need to know what the scoring system is.

## Case studies

Case studies, if written properly are frequently self-explanatory, but it is common to use them as part of a larger, sometimes more formal session. If used in isolation, for example to form the basis of a discussion or teaching session, then this needs to be explained at the beginning. If used as part of a group work exercise, then the guidelines given below should be used. In any case, the scenarios and activities should be read through and if necessary, explained as part of the introduction.

## Group work

Generally, the introduction should include details of the work to be investigated, information about time constraints, the division of the larger group into smaller ones (if appropriate), and an explanation of how the work will be monitored. If the group is to work on a problem in depth and over a longer period of time, then the students, during the introduction, can outline the results of their preliminary reading and investigations.

# Development

The development of the session should contain the major part of the information (if teacher-centred), or the major part of the activity (if student-centred). It is during this time that themes will be unfolded, relationships should hopefully develop, and the subject area is explored in more depth. Below are some brief guidelines for each of the methods being discussed.

## Lecture

If looking at a particular problem, such as child abuse, during the development phase, the nature of the problem should be expanded, and if more informal methods are being used, then it is at this time that the students' ideas should be developed and integrated into the session. Following this, the possible solutions to the particular problem should either be presented or formulated with the group.

To ensure symmetry and closure are maintained, the problem should again be restated, and the appropriate solutions applied.

If the subject in hand is not particularly problem based, then the development stage should be used as an expansion period where the topic is built around a set of key points given in the introduction. For example, in the introduction to a session on a disease, some key facts regarding its nature, aetiology, effects and prognosis can be given.

It is a good idea, in order to captivate interest to include (at the beginning) some unusual facts such as "cystic fibrosis was first described over 2000 years ago, although not recognised by medical science until the first part of this century". In the development, the theme can then be expanded to its discovery during a heat wave in New York and the effect it was having on sufferers, and how the original diagnosis was made. Following this, the use of sweat tests can be explained.

## Demonstration

The development of the demonstration can be divided into student and teacher activities. As far as the teacher-centred activities are concerned, the procedure should be worked through at the normal speed, and then worked through at a slower pace, putting emphasis on each skill involved.

The students should then be able, under supervision, to practise the technique. This may be done either by allowing them to carry out the procedure without comment first and giving feedback at the end, or by supervising them as they go through it.

## Seminar

The development of the seminar will naturally share many of the characteristics of the lecture and discussion methods. At the end of each component of the seminar, the facilitator of the session should briefly review what has been said, and link it into the next part of the session.

## Discussion

During the development stage, the following points should be followed.

1. Formulate topic areas with appropriate questions and prompts.
2. Take notes throughout the discussion in order to form the summary.
3. Ensure the physical environment is conducive to discussion.
4. If necessary, introduce confidentiality rules.

The role of the discussion leader is to

1. Prompt, but not dominate.
2. Encourage comments by praise and respect all contributions.
3. Summarise and interpret unclear contributions.

When using "structured controversy" (e.g. Pederson, 1992), small groups of students are given the brief to argue a viewpoint of a topic forcefully, whilst another group has to formulate an argument against it. This may be reversed.

## Role play

The development stage of the role play method is for the students to act out the identified roles within an agreed framework. The role of the facilitator at this stage is naturally dependent on the constraints put upon the participants at the beginning of the session. For instance, the role play may be free ranging so that it leads to a natural conclusion with a free expression of emotions. In this case the facilitator's role will be to ensure the emotional safety of participants and to intercede if the activity gets out of hand. If the role play is to be confined to exploring a much narrower area such as admitting a patient, then the facilitator is responsible for ensuring that the activity achieves that goal.

## Simulations/games

The development stage with these methods is obviously highly experiential and comprises the students actually carrying out the activity. The role of the facilitator here is to act as a referee, ensuring that rules are obeyed and, in the case of games, that points are correctly awarded. In the case of simulations such as those for cardiopulmonary resuscitation, the facilitator's role at this stage may be that of an informed preceptor to guide participants through the experience and also to offer support if needed.

## Case studies

Since case studies may be undertaken individually or in groups, the role of the facilitator has to be adapted accordingly. It is fairly common that if undertaken individually, then the student may wish to discuss points as they encounter them. Hence more formal questions at the end of the case study could be redundant. If used as part of group work, then the guidelines given below should be utilised.

## Group work

The purpose of the development stage of group work is essentially to generate ideas, generate solutions or to analyse critically. It may of course be a combination of all three. The role of the facilitator therefore, must be partly as an expert providing advice and guidance and also as a catalyst to promote problem solving and ideas. Although the purposes of group work appear rather far-reaching, it should be remembered that it relies heavily on the student's experiences, attitudes and in terms of cooperative learning strategies, communication skills.

## Conclusions

The conclusions to teacher-centred approaches will be geared to drawing together the information presented in order to complete the symmetrical pattern of the the session. By doing so, it is hoped that the reiteration of vital points will encourage learning and also that for some students, closure will occur.

In student-centred approaches, the conclusions will form a vital part of the learning process in so far as they will integrate the deliberations and reflections of the group into a meaningful outcome which can be utilised by participants. Without an effective conclusion, activities such as group work will have little meaning.

*Lecture*

Summarise main points and for informal lecture methods, integrate results of facilitator/ student interactions, perhaps to the point of dispelling misconceptions that have arisen during the session. For both formal and informal sessions, further references should be made available so that students can investigate the topic further.

*Demonstration*

The conclusions to the demonstration method will largely depend on what the demonstration was about. It may take the form of student questions and answers or it may be appropriate to end the session with the student demonstrating the skill themselves. Ethically, it must encompass the question of competence, further practice required and supervision that may be needed.

*Seminar*

The conclusions to a seminar can, if the facilitator has not been active throughout the session, be incomplete and meaningless. The conclusions should include not only a brief summary of the formal parts of the session, as mentioned above, but also the salient point arising from discussion (see below).

*Discussion*

Throughout the session, the facilitator should have been noting points that have been raised by the group. If these have not been clear at the time, then clarification should have been sought, usually by rephrasing the point and asking the participants for confirmation. If this has been done, then the conclusions can comprise the main subject areas that have been raised and a synopsis of the discussion that ensued.

*Role play*

The conclusions following role play are very different from other methods. They comprise the facilitator exploring the individual's feeling about the situation and generating discussion to explore how this relates to real life; in other words how they will be able to use what they have gained in their own practice. It is crucial that the facilitator de-roles all individuals in the group and particularly if the role play has been about a very emotive subject, to offer individual counselling where necessary.

*Simulations/games*

The role of the facilitator where a game has been completed is, apart from announcing the winner, to ensure that the group is able to draw conclusions from the game that it can relate to practice. So this conclusion will take the form of a discussion, with the facilitator asking for and giving examples, exploring problems and identifying solutions.

Simulations will help to identify both merits and deficits in practice within a safe environment. During the conclusion stage of this session, in-depth reflection may be essential either on an individual or group basis in order to assess the implications for future clinical practice.

## Case studies

The feedback from the points raised by the individual or group will form the basis of the conclusions. It is often necessary to add the facilitator's expert perspectives to the final discussion. It is common for further areas of development to be identified at this stage.

## Group work

If the culmination of the group work has been a general discussion, then the guidelines given for concluding a discussion should be followed. If, however, student presentation either verbally or on charts has occurred then a similar format should be followed with consensus, sharing and reflection forming the basis of the conclusion.

# Conclusions

Prescriptive teaching strategies are not particularly useful when considered as unique and inflexible entities. Although several methods have been described in this chapter, it is likely that most preceptors will adapt them to suit their own teaching style. This will often take the form of incorporating two or three different strategies in one session and this is not only acceptable but advisable in order to enhance student motivation.

Although the outline has suggested some functions of the teacher at each stage, it is recommended that the taxonomy posed by Steinaker and Bell (1979) be used to further define the role in any given situation.

# Summary

One way of looking at the role of the teacher and the strategies that may be used is to consider the type of learning that will occur, and this in turn is usually dependent on the subject matter and students (Steinaker and Bell, 1979). In this experiential learning theory, Steinaker and Bell organise learning into the following taxonomy: exposure; participation; identification; internalisation; dissemination.

Some authors (e.g. Dux, 1989) have urged teachers to examine their motives in choosing a particular method.

The level of the material presented is quite naturally an important factor, but perhaps more important are the abilities of the students to cope with the information.

The lecture, despite being teacher-centred, is one of the more popular methods favoured by both students and teachers (Dux, 1989). Although a period of questions and answers should be included at the end of a formal lecture, if this is the sole method of teaching, a more advisable strategy is to use the informal lecture method where student–preceptor interaction is encouraged throughout.

The seminar is, typically, a combination of formal exposition and discussion and can be used for sessions where a series of papers is to be presented, different aspects of care are to be covered or even where students have reviewed the literature on a subject and wish to present it in a structured way.

The demonstration involves, by its very nature, a "visual explanation of facts, concepts and procedures" (Quinn, 1988).

A discussion format can be used effectively to help students to understand concepts that may have been covered in a previous session, as a debriefing exercise to other strategies, or just to explore facets of a topic, particularly where personal experiences and attitudes may help others to learn.

Role play is used most frequently when the preceptor wants the students to be able to empathise with a particular group of people.

A simulation is essentially an extended role play with structure and rules.

Games can vary from a simulation where individuals are in competition with each other, to board- and computer-based games which may have one or multiple participants.

Case studies can be used either as a teaching or assessment strategy, and facilitate problem solving.

Quite apart from the motivational aspects of group work, these methods are used to improve communication, foster cooperation between students, provide peer support and of course to share ideas. In achieving this it is hoped to facilitate problem solving and critical thinking.

Generally most sessions can be divided up into introduction, development and conclusions.

# References

Baldwin, D., Hill, P. and Hanson, G. (1991) Performance of psychomotor skills: a comparison of two teaching strategies. *Journal of Nursing Education* **30**(8), 367–370.

Burnard, P. and Morrison, P. (1991) Preferred teaching and learning strategies. *Nursing Times*, **87**(38), 52.

Curzon, L.B. (1990) *Teaching in Further Education: an outline of Principles and Practice*. **4th edn**. London: Cassell.

Dux, C.M. (1989) An investigation into whether nurse teachers take into account the individual learning styles of their students when formulating teaching strategies. *Nurse Education Today*, **9**, 186–191.

Felder, B.J. (1992) Using a game format to improve compliance with required review of hospital standards and policies. *Journal of Continuing Education in Nursing*, **23**(5), 209–211.

Frisch, N. (1987) Cognitive Maturity of nursing students. *Journal of Nursing Scholarship*, **19**, 25–27.

Johnson, D.W. and Johnson, R.T (1988) Critical thinking through structured controversy. *Educational Leadership*, **45**(8), 58–63.

Klaassens, E. (1992) Strategies to enhance problem solving. *Nurse Educator*, **17**(3), 28–30.

Pederson, C. (1992) Effects of structured controversy on students' perceptions of their skills in discussing controversial issues. *Journal of Nursing Education*, **31** (3), 101–106.

Quinn, F.M. (1988) *The Principles and Practice of Nurse Education*, 2nd edn. Croom Helm.

Steinaker, N. and Bell, M. (1979) *The Experiential Taxonomy: a New Approach to Teaching and Learning*. New York: Academic Press.

# chapter eight

# The clinical learning environment

## Introduction

Theories of teaching and learning go a long way to telling us how the individual may effectively learn, but they are by no means infallible in terms of their effectiveness in predicting learning outcomes. Earlier chapters have examined some of the factors that affect learning, such as memory, attention, perception and motivation. Even if we take these factors into account, learning may still be impaired by other factors which come under the collective term of "learning environment".

It is difficult to give an all-embracing definition of what is meant by a learning environment. Principally, as Quinn (1988) points out when describing the clinical learning environment, it is "a holistic notion involving every aspect of a clinical setting involving the students themselves". It is perhaps an impossible task, especially when considering the fact that much learning is interactive, to distinguish completely between outside factors such as the mentor, preceptor, systems used within the workplace, etc., and the individual's reactions to them.

If we accept that in some form the learning environment is a tangible concept, and that as such it can be measured, then we need to give some thought to the possibilities and implications of a relevant audit system. This will be discussed not in isolation, but rather with its natural partner, namely quality assurance, in order to give us some idea as to the standards that we must work towards.

The discussion will begin by examining briefly one of the most basic conditions required for learning to take place, namely motivation, and it will be seen that the learning environment itself is an interactive concept between the individual and outside factors.

## Motivation and need theory

In identifying human needs, Maslow (1970) has postulated that some will remain relatively unimportant until certain other needs have been satisfied; hence the hierarchical nature of his model (Figure 8.1). The implications for the learning environment, and more specifically to individuals is briefly explored below.

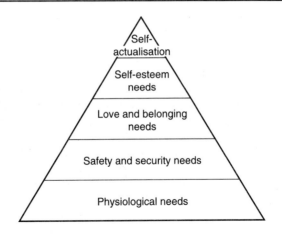

**Figure 8.1.** Hierarchy of human needs (Maslow, 1970).

## Physiological needs

Although not normally associated with learning, this particular area does have an important role to play. Basic requirements such as having enough money to provide an adequate diet, living accommodation, and even the pressure of study causing sleep disturbances, are all important personal factors in determining how much learning will take place. Fatigue brought about through excessive travelling or even a hectic social life are well known to most of us and will eventually take their toll.

## Towards security

We are all aware of our need to feel secure and to have a sense of belonging in our personal lives and to the individual who is attempting to learn, these needs are just as important. The need for security is of particular concern in nursing where students move from area to area on a regular basis and frequently do not become a part of the ward team.

This, however, presents us with only half of the picture because, naturally, even whilst working in a ward area, particularly during long shifts, students often form affiliations with peers in preference to trained staff.

The need for security can be difficult to fulfil in the clinical environment for the learner, and yet Maslow emphasises its importance as second only to the basic physiological needs in his hierarchy. If we are to create an effective learning environment, we must therefore consider how best we can make the learner feel secure.

Perhaps the key to providing a secure environment lies in the sister/charge nurse being seen by the student as being responsible for controlling the clinical learning environment (Orton, 1981), although such a statement must not be made without analysing the possible reasons for it. Certainly in terms of learning, a climate conducive to integrating new information should be achieved, and it could be argued that this presents security in itself by ensuring continuity with the other facets of the student's world, i.e. ensuring that theory and practice are integrated.

The following strategies may be used in order to facilitate the student's perception of security:

1. Ensure that the teaching methods employed are in accordance with what the student perceives as the most effective learning method (Burnard and Morrison, 1991). It appears that students favour more structured teacher-centred approaches, whilst those responsible for teaching nurses seem to favour students organising and carrying out their own learning sessions. Naturally the quality of student-centred learning method used is of paramount importance, although it should be said that threatening experiences, e.g. carrying out procedures when the student perceives their knowledge is inadequate, rarely help anyone to learn, and only increase the student's feelings of insecurity.

2. Reduce potential role conflict by ensuring that student nurses are not given instructions contrary to what they have been taught (Jones, 1978). This has been identified as a major source of stress, and close cooperation between nurse teachers and clinical staff is vital.

3. Ensure a comprehensive orientation programme as anxiety is often related to the initial part of the clinical experience (Sellek, 1978). It should be ensured that individual needs are identified at the beginning of the experience.

4. To reduce potential anxiety, it is important to ensure that students are well supported when caring for patients who are terminally ill (Birch, 1979).

5. Having an identified mentor/preceptor responsible for individual students will help to reduce initial anxiety (see Chapter four), provided, of course that a degree of autonomy on the part of the student in choosing a mentor, is allowed.

6. Ensure, whenever possible, that the student has peer support.

It is often the case, as with student-centred learning, that the students themselves may feel under threat and that theories of teaching and learning which, in ideal conditions are effective, may, under certain circumstances have the opposite effect.

As a final word of caution to this short discussion on security, it is not helpful make direct comparisons between individuals, especially when one of those individuals is a mentor or preceptor and the other is a student. The only way to ascertain how an individual feels is, by gaining their trust, to allow them to express themselves. The individual who feels insecure will normally show reluctance to embark on a course of action where the outcome is not certain, and this of course is entirely normal. This can be largely overcome by a trusting relationship with a more senior member of staff, in which doubts, fears and deficiencies in knowledge can be freely expressed.

## Towards a feeling of belonging

In terms of Maslow's theory, it is difficult to see, particularly in relation to short allocations to a clinical area, how a true sense of belonging can be fostered. Naturally, making the student feel valued and part of the team, if only in a relatively minor capacity, will go some way to achieving this.

As has already been mentioned, peer contact will often form the basis of feelings of security, particularly in the early part of the education process, and this may lead to a sense of belonging.

In the more general sense, however, the student member of a team should be made to feel that they have something useful to contribute, and whereas purely observational experiences are sometimes very useful and almost certainly unavoidable, they should be combined with a degree of involvement, even if this is only seeking and valuing their opinions and reflections.

## Self-esteem

The people in the learning environment will be instrumental in making the student feel good about themselves and the contributions that they make. Generally speaking, high self-esteem will come about when the individual feels that they are valued by others and that they are an important part of the team. Personal experiences, opinions and even concerns, if dealt with properly can all serve to increase the student's self-esteem. Conversely, feeling as though they are "in the way", inexperienced and alone, quite apart from detracting from a sense of belonging and making them feel insecure, may also lead to a deterioration in self-esteem.

## Self-actualisation

The pinnacle of human achievement is viewed by humanist psychologists as *self-actualisation*. It is characterised by a need for "goodness" with all that entails with our relationship with the world around us. The individual who self-actualises, for instance tolerates uncertainty, appreciates other people unconditionally and generally accepts their circumstances. Naturally, the individual will need to have the lower needs fulfilled before reaching this point, and Maslow is emphatic that few individuals ever reach this stage.

# The clinical area as a learning environment

As with any profession, the workplace for which the individual is being educated to work in is of vital importance to the amount and quality of learning that takes place.

## Clinical personnel

The role of mentors and preceptors has been discussed elsewhere in the text, although it is appropriate to revisit this topic briefly for the purposes of this discussion. In considering the learning environment as being partly the product of interactions between certain key individuals, it is perhaps relevant to examine the effects this may have.

In examining the learning environment, many authors have placed an emphasis on the ward sister as being perceived by students as being instrumental in creating and controlling the climate in which learning takes place (e.g. Fretwell, 1980; Orton, 1981). Where such a structure exists, it would indeed seem logical to deduce that such a key managerial and clinical position would have such an effect; however, Fretwell (1979) points out that, amongst other things, a hierarchical structure may actually be detrimental to learning, although this may be overcome by effective teamwork, negotiation and effective communication.

The nurse teacher attached to the unit should be able not only to add in some instances to the clinical expertise resource for the student, but also to act as a resource for staff involved in preceptorship and mentoring. The student will also have been allocated a personal tutor who will normally be outside of that particular clinical area. The role of the personal tutor may vary considerably from one college to another, and indeed the discussion on mentorship and preceptorship is as relevant to this role as it is to clinically based education. Suffice it to say that the personal tutor may assist with such matters as study skills, personal difficulties and individual academic tuition as well as acting as a valuable resource for the student.

Quite naturally, as health care is a multidisciplinary concept, other members of the health care team such as medical staff, physiotherapists and occupational therapists, will also be part of the learning environment.

## Role-modelling

The organisational aspect of the learning environment should not be viewed as a separate entity. The organisation of learning experiences which are to be effective must be a multifaceted exercise in terms of interpersonal contacts, especially if it is accepted that a significant amount of learning occurs through "role-modelling".

Marson (1981) emphasises that effective teachers in the clinical situation are perceived by learners as having an attitude of care and concern for the welfare of others as well as having a commitment to the education of students in particular. Other authors (e.g. Ogier, 1989), have also emphasised the role-modelling component of learning. If we acknowledge that learning will take place as a result of role modelling, then we should examine some key areas that will determine its effectiveness.

## Person-to-person conflict

Although a subject of much debate and diverse theories, it is worthwhile mentioning that there are times when people just do not get on with each other! The reasons can be many and varied; it may be differences of temperament, beliefs, attitudes – the list is almost endless. In earlier chapters, the advisability of the student choosing their own mentor has been discussed, and this may overcome many potential difficulties.

As a general rule, it should be borne in mind that just as role-modelling may occur if the conditions are right for it to do so, so the student may miss learning opportunities or reject certain behaviours purely because they do not like the individual who exhibits them.

## Clinical competence and expertise

It is a natural consequence of our discussion that the learning environment can only be effective if those personnel involved in it are well informed and clinically competent. It was mentioned earlier that both clinical and college staff should be teaching in a non-conflicting way. Updating personal knowledge should not merely be a "re-registering" exercise, but should be linked to practice, and should be an ongoing activity. The advent of the Framework and Higher Award gives nurses the opportunity to link learning directly with clinical practice.

## Resources

The resources that any clinical area may have extend far beyond just journals and textbooks. The whole subject of audio-visual aids is covered elsewhere in the text, but for the purposes of our discussion here, a short list of possible resources is given. It will be noticed that a significant resource area can be developed for relatively little cost, and it is advisable to have a specific area set aside for such resources, and most certainly to have a named person responsible for it, perhaps on a rota basis.

1. *Journals*. Collected either from individuals who take particular journals on a regular basis, or by ward/unit subscriptions. Some discussion with ward/unit staff about the selection of these journals is essential in order to ensure their most effective use.
2. *Textbooks*. Find out whether there is a fund from which the finance for textbooks can be provided. Care needs to be taken to avoid hoarding (and hence probable use of) out-of-date/irrelevant texts.
3. *References*. There are several ways to build up a bank of relevant references. One possible way is for a member of staff to be delegated each month to scan the appropriate journals and to record a brief abstract of each one which could then form the basis of a reference section.
4. *Product information*. Manufacturers' information about their products which are being used in the clinical area is vital. Drugs, appliances and equipment will all have information relating to their use, as well as (in many cases) published research which justifies its use. All this information could be held centrally in a resource area.
5. *External agencies*. Information from self-help groups, national organisations and even relevant government agencies which may be applicable to the client group.
6. *Health education literature*. This is a superb resource which is readily available and usually free of charge.
7. *Projects and local research*. These may have been carried out by members of staff as part of a course, or by past students or medical staff.
8. *Department information*. Outlining the services offered by other departments in the hospital.
9. *Contact names*. Staff throughout the unit (or indeed outside) who are useful resources to the student (e.g. environmental health, dietician.).

# Education audit of the clinical learning environment

As already stated in the introduction, the clinical learning environment must be considered as a tangible entity, and as such, must be audited as a vital component of the overall education process. It comes as no surprise therefore that such an audit is a requirement of the course submission (ENB, 1990) in order that students are allowed to gain experience within that clinical area.

The approach that can be taken towards this subject can be geared towards participating either in an existing audit system or in developing a combined quality assurance/audit system as described below.

Although it has been said that the system combines quality assurance with an audit, this is in fact somewhat misleading, as the two concepts are inextricably linked. If a clinical area is being audited, then a measurable standard must be used in order to indicate whether aspects of that environment are satisfactory or unsatisfactory. It is for this reason that a brief explanation of the concept of quality is given below.

# Quality assurance defined

The use of quality assurance tools in the clinical environment is now becoming a more familiar phenomenon although, due to the usage of generic systems such as "Monitor", and "QUALPACS", many nurses will not have had the experience of constructing a system of their own. The use of auditing systems in education, whether in the classroom or in the clinical environment, will follow the same basic principles.

Firstly, however, it is useful to define quality as a starting point, and the definition given below provides us with a sufficiently generic approach:

> The measurement of the actual level of the service provided plus the efforts to modify when necessary the provision of these services in the light of the results of these measurements. (Williamson, 1982).

As with any area of any practice which attempts to evaluate the effectiveness of a particular system, the starting point is to devise a model (or adapt an existing one) so that we may have a basic framework with which to proceed. The model described below (Maxwell, 1984) has been seen as traditionally of use in the more familiar context of quality assessment in health. Bassett (1993), in examining Maxwell's model, has found that with adaptation it can be applied to nurse education.

# Maxwell's model of quality

Maxwell (1984) identifies six dimensions in health care:

1. Access to services.
2. Relevance to need.
3. Effectiveness.
4. Equity.
5. Social acceptability.
6. Efficiency and economy.

In terms of the use for which this model was originally intended, the standards which will be applicable under each of the above dimensions will quite naturally be geared directly towards patient care, and will be dependent on how each one of the dimensions has been defined. Therefore, if we are to adapt the model effectively, then we need to redefine them. Bassett (1993), in looking at nurse education has redefined them as follows:

> *Access to services*. Flexibility of tutors working hours to allow access by students for a longer period each day.
> *Relevance to need*. Liaison with service managers/purchasing health authorities, e.g. ensuring that an adequate number of nurses are produced for each branch area.
> *Effectiveness*. Identifying which teaching methods are most effective and in which situations.
> *Equity*. Fair division of the budget between the various courses.
> *Social acceptability*. Acceptability of the college by students, staff and purchasing authorities.
> *Efficiency and economy*. Projected student costs must be accurate and competitive whilst maintaining high quality.

Naturally the above dimensions have been defined by Bassett in terms of the non-clinical learning environment (the college). What we have to do now is to examine these dimensions in terms of the clinical learning environment. In considering the example definitions below, the reader can extend them and make them more specific to their own area of practice.

*Access to services*. Availability of mentors, preceptors and resources to the student.
*Relevance to need*. Compatibility of clinical practice with student/curriculum learning outcomes.
*Effectiveness*. Effective learning facilitated through appropriate strategies by professionally credible preceptors.
*Equity*. Equality for all students, within the context of curricular and personal objectives, of experience and opportunity.
*Social acceptability*. Compatibility of clinical experience with student, college and national requirements.
*Efficiency and economy*. Uniform, economic and high quality integration of practice and education.

## Standard setting

Having completed the above exercise, the next step in this process is to develop standards for each of the key words or phrases. Naturally, this is normally a function of a quality circle following extensive consultation with colleagues. It is relevant here though to pause briefly in order to examine the meaning of a standard statement and then to examine a method by which they can be classified.

## *Definitions* (RCN, 1990)

*Standard*. Professionally agreed level of performance for a particular population which is achievable, observable, desirable and measurable.
*Standard statement*. A statement which describes the broad objectives of your standard.
*Structure criteria*. These relate to resources in the system which are necessary for the successful completion of the task/area under review.
*Process criteria*. These relate to actions undertaken by tutorial staff in conjunction with students, service managers, etc.
*Outcome criteria*. These relate to the desired effect of, e.g. education in terms of student behaviours, responses, level of knowledge and application of that knowledge.

The process described, by its very nature, does not permit short cuts to be taken but nevertheless some basic and fundamental errors do occur. Firstly, the standards are not validated within the area in question and hence are not appropriate. Secondly, consensus regarding the content of statements is minimal or absent, leading to conflicting practice. Thirdly, the process may be viewed from too narrow a perspective and may not take into account key personnel in an effective way. Naturally setting up an effective consultative process will overcome the first two difficulties.

One way of overcoming the third difficulty is to gather data from a variety of sources, e.g. the student, the mentor, the education staff and the clinical managers. Most common now is the practice of utilising student questionnaires about clinical placements. The practice of verbal discussions following clinical activity as a sole source of evaluation has been criticised (Beech, 1991) as being "negatively phrased and detached". It would seem logical therefore that, particularly within the context of being able to form direct comparisons based on some form of standard criteria, a questionnaire approach would be appropriate in most circumstances. The Delphi method has been used to evaluate clinical experiences with some success. This is a method which has been adapted from a system used to evaluate classroom sessions. The reader is referred to ENB (1987) where a full discussion of the method is provided.

The participation of students in the auditing process can actually be achieved by more than one route, firstly, as has been discussed, by the completion of questionnaires. These questionnaires may be fairly non-specific to the clinical area and may be directed primarily towards the quality of the learning environment; they may also include items such as systems for delivery of care. In rather rarer circumstances it may be geared towards more specific clinical aspects of the area. Secondly, there should be a student input into the audit system described above. Thirdly, there should be student participation in the curriculum planning process which should ideally be based on quantifiable information.

# Summary

The need for security is of particular concern in nursing where students move from area to area on a regular basis and frequently do not become a part of the ward team.

Students often form affiliations with peers in preference to trained staff (Reid *et al.*, 1991).

The following strategies may be used in order to facilitate the students perception of security:

1. Ensure that the teaching methods employed are in accordance with what the student perceives as the most effective learning method (Burnard and Morrison, 1991).
2. Reduce potential role conflict by ensuring that student nurses are not given instructions contrary to what they have been taught (Jones, 1978).
3. Ensure a comprehensive orientation programme as anxiety is often related to the initial part of the clinical experience (Sellek, 1978).
4. To reduce potential anxiety, it is important to ensure that students are well supported when caring for patients who are terminally ill (Birch, 1979).
5. Having an identified mentor/preceptor responsible for individual students will help to reduce initial anxiety.
6. Ensure, whenever possible, that the student has peer support.

The student member of a team should be made to feel that they have something useful to contribute.

Fretwell (1979) points out that, amongst other things, a hierarchical structure may actually be detrimental to learning, although this may be overcome by effective teamwork, negotiation and effective communication.

The nurse teacher attached to the unit should be able not only to add in some instances to the clinical expertise resource for the student, but also to act as a resource for staff involved in preceptorship and mentoring.

Marson (1981) emphasises that effective teachers in the clinical situation are perceived by learners as having an attitude of care and concern for the welfare of others as well as having a commitment to the education of students in particular.

The clinical learning environment must be considered as a tangible entity, and as such, must be audited as a vital component of the overall education process.

Maxwell identifies six dimensions in health care:

1. Access to services.
2. Relevance to need.

3. Effectiveness.
4. Equity.
5. Social acceptability.
6. Efficiency and economy.

A "standard" is a professionally agreed level of performance for a particular population which is achievable, observable, desirable and measurable.

A "standard statement" describes the broad objectives of your standard.

"Structure criteria" relate to resources in the system which are necessary for the successful completion of the task/area under review.

"Process criteria" relate to actions undertaken by tutorial staff in conjunction with students, service managers, etc.

"Outcome criteria" relate to the desired effect of, e.g. education in terms of student behaviours, responses, level of knowledge and application of that knowledge.

# Related activities

## Activity 1

Using the definitions given below, and, if required adding to them, write up to five key words or phrases that typify the dimensions e.g.: Access to Services: availability of staff, flexibility of service, resources, support.

Access to services.
Relevance to need.
Effectiveness.
Equity.
Social Acceptability.
Efficiency and economy.

## Activity 2

Using one of the key words/phrases from Activity 1, write a standard using the four criteria below:

Standard statement.
Structure criteria.
Process criteria.
Outcome criteria.

# References

Bassett, C.C. (1993) Quality assurance in nurse education. *Nurse Education Today*, 13, 55–59.

Beech, B.F. (1991) Changes: The Delphi technique adapted for classroom evaluation of clinical placements. *Nurse Education Today*, 11, 207–212.

Birch, J. (1979) The anxious learners. *Nursing Mirror*, 148(6), 17–22.

Burnard, P. and Morrison, P. (1991) Preferred teaching and learning strategies. *Nursing Times*, 87(38), 52.

ENB (1990) Regulations and guidelines for the approval of institutions and courses.

Fretwell, J.E. (1979) Socialisation of nurses: teaching and learning in hospital wards. Thesis, Warwick University.

Fretwell, J.E. (1980) An enquiry into the ward learning environment. *Nursing Times*, **76**, 26. (Occasional Paper 69-75.)

Jones, D. (1978) The need for a comprehensive counselling service for nursing students. *Journal of Advanced Nursing*, **13**(4), 359–368.

Marson, S.N. (1981) Ward teaching skills—An investigation into the behavioural characteristics of effective ward teachers. Thesis, CNAA Sheffield City Polytechnic.

Maslow, A. (1970) *Motivation and Personality*, 2nd edn. New York: Harper and Row.

Maxwell, R.J. (1984) Quality assessment in health. *British Medical Journal*. 12 May, 288.

Ogier, M.E. (1989) *Working and Learning: The Learning Environment in Clinical Nursing*. London: Scutari.

Orton, H.D. (1981) Ward learning climates and student nurse responses. *Nursing Times*, **77**, 23. (Occasional Paper 65-68.)

Quinn, F.M. (1988) *The Principles and Practice of Nurse Education*. 2nd edn. London: Chapman and Hall.

RCN (1990) *The Dynamic Standard Setting System: RCN Standards of Care Project*. Harrow, Middlesex: Scutari Projects.

Sellek, T. (1978) Satisfying and anxiety-creating incidents as identified by student nurses during the process of becoming an SRN. Thesis, Manchester University.

# chapter nine

# The process of assessment

## Introduction

The subject of assessment involves factors which relate to how an individual learns, how an individual puts his/her learning into practice and even the psychological and logistical factors involved in attempting to ascertain how much learning has taken place. On first inspection of the subject, assessment would appear to be quite simple, in that if learning has occurred then it must, in some way or another, stand up to some form of assessment. In reality, many questions need to be asked about the techniques used in assessment and the assumptions that underlie them, and this cannot be tackled in isolation from the assumptions which underlie the theories of learning used, experiences available and indeed the very philosophy of the curriculum.

Learning, as has already been discussed, is not an altogether straightforward process and, by implication, neither is assessment. For example, in trying to ascertain the degree of competence in communicating with a patient, attitudes, communication skills, environment and personality will all have an effect on the outcome. The central question that needs to be addressed is that of which factors can be assessed and which factors cannot. To return to our discussion in an earlier chapter, the assessment strategy for a skills-based course would be rather different from that of a predominantly student-centred course where the learning outcomes are that much broader.

The trend away from periodic practice-based assessments to continuous assessment (ENB, 1988) to some extent reflects the complexities both of the learning process and of the nature of nursing itself. Conversely, the requirement that nurses should meet certain competencies will also add another dimension to the subject. As has already been mentioned, to follow one school of thought stringently with regard to the nature of learning is perhaps unwise, bearing in mind the vast array of competencies which need to be mastered. The types of assessment which can be used are varied and range from journal keeping to formal written examinations. The purposes of such assessments are naturally just as varied, but within our discussion, the general classifications of "Formative" and "Summative" will be explored.

## Formative and summative assessments

The terms *formative* and *summative* are possibly the most widely used terms in assessment. There is a tendency to treat them as distinct entities and to classify assessments into one or the other accordingly. Broadly speaking, formative assessment refers to the process of ascertaining a student's progress during a course of study or experience, usually in an informal way. It is usually individually-based and will not normally be counted towards a final mark or grade. It is reasonable to suggest that such assessments not only will lead to the student gaining an insight into their areas of strengths and weaknesses in a non-threatening manner, but also should guide further learning strategies. By implication, the outcome of formative assessments may occasionally direct both the student and the teacher to the conclusion that the student has little aptitude for the subject, and hence counselling may be required.

Summative assessment, on the other hand, involves the assessment of learning which has taken place and hopefully applied to practice and is most obviously typified by a final examination (usually written).

Both types of assessment have their roles to play. The formative assessment essentially allows us to "diagnose" difficulties and, with the student, to "prescribe" corrective action. The summative assessment is traditionally a far more decisive tool and will always have a strong bearing on the individual's future within that course of study. There is however, an alternative way of considering these two types of assessment. Instead of considering them as separate entities, it has been suggested (Rowntree, 1977) that they are opposite ends of a continuum with uniquely formative and summative assessments occurring relatively rarely. Most assessments therefore can be seen as having an element of each to some extent. For example, most formative assessments will therefore contribute towards decisions regarding the individual's future and most summative assessments, particularly if effective feedback is given, will act as a diagnostic tool which will direct further learning.

The assessment continuum can be depicted as follows:

Formative   . . . . . . . . . . . . . . . . . . . . .   Summative

(Diagonal Line)

Rowntree (1977) further went on to identify other continuum to describe further types of assessment.

| | | |
|---|---|---|
| Informal | . . . . . . . . . . . . . . . . . . . . . | Formal |
| Process | . . . . . . . . . . . . . . . . . . . . . | Product |
| Divergent | . . . . . . . . . . . . . . . . . . . . . | Convergent |
| Idiographic | . . . . . . . . . . . . . . . . . . . . . | Nomothetic |
| Course Work | . . . . . . . . . . . . . . . . . . . . . | Examinations |
| Continuous | . . . . . . . . . . . . . . . . . . . . . | Terminal |

*Informal–formal.* Formal assessment aims to gain knowledge about the student but essentially has no instructional value. Informal assessment, on the other hand, is diagnostic and should be unobtrusive. Rowntree describes formal assessment as "publicly satisfied purpose for public use" and informal as "privately specific purpose for private use". Individual formative tutorials are examples of an informal assessment.

*Process–product.* A process assessment through techniques such as projects, student-centred learning and contract learning, reveals how a student has learned, whereas a product assessment will merely reveal the end result of the process.

*Divergent–convergent.* Divergent assessment is, by necessity, individually tailored because it examines the individual's development in contrast to the convergent assessment (typically a final standard examination) which tells the assessor more about the similarities between students rather than the ways in which they diverge. Certain project work could be said to be divergent but only if the individual is allowed to explore and investigate in an individual manner.

*Idiographic–nomothetic.* Student-centred and self-assessment techniques can be said to be idiographic in so far as they attempt to discover the uniqueness of the individual. Nomothetic assessments are concerned with a more standardised form of data collection from the process, (marking, streaming, etc.).

*Course Work–exams.* According to Rowntree a summative assessment at the end of the course cannot be justified without information regarding the work that has been completed throughout the course. Naturally both course work and examinations may take many forms and here the grey areas between formative and summative are most evident.

*Continuous–terminal.* Although continuous assessment is an admirable tool for formative aspects of the process, it will usually contribute to a final summative grade. Traditionally in nursing (ENB, 1987), a terminal examination is required although it could be argued that if an acceptable summative assessment could be compiled from the continuous assessment tool then terminal examination would not be necessary.

On examination of these various types of assessment, it is feasible that the items on the left-hand side are components of, and interact with, each other. For instance, a formative assessment could be said to be informal, process based, divergent, ideographic, continuous and established through course work. Conversely, a summative assessment could be said to be formal, product based, convergent, nomothetic, unique and concerned with terminal or periodic exams.

The discussion on formative and summative assessment is central to this chapter and will be revisited later in terms of assessment strategy and the guidelines within which they must operate. The next stage in the discussion will be centred upon the question of how far we can depend on the results of an assessment to give us the information we require accurately.

# Validity

Validity can be said to be "an examination of the approximate truth or falsity of the propositions" (Cook and Campbell, 1979). Put more simply it is "a measure of the truth or accuracy of a claim" (Burns and Grove, 1987). In terms of assessment, it could be adjusted to ask the question: "Do we believe that the results reflect accurately what is purported to have been tested?" Many questions will surround the debate concerning validity and many of these questions have their foundation in learning theory. For instance, can the student actually carry out the nursing care that they have written about in the final examination or did they learn it by rote? Does the assessment reflect what the student actually does or will do or does it reflect their ability to take an assessment?

Broadly speaking, validity, as with research, can be divided into five categories:

1. *Face validity.* This type of validity is highly informal and to an extent instinctive in as far as it is concerned with whether the assessment looks as though it will reveal the relevant information. It is only possible realistically in the light of professional knowledge, expertise and an in-depth understanding of the other types of validity.
2. *Construct validity.* This refers to how the assessment is constructed in terms of pass/fail criteria, progression of knowledge, formative and summative components as well as procedural implications such as examination boards and regulations.
3. *Content validity.* This refers to what is actually being assessed and not only refers to items such as competencies but also addresses the question about whether items can realistically be assessed or not (e.g. attitudes).
4. *Concurrent validity.* Ideally, if an assessment is to reveal useful information we need to

know to what extent this can be done. This is difficult with an entirely new assessment strategy and hence it needs to be based substantially on either the results of similar strategies elsewhere or the results of pilot schemes.

5. *Predictive validity*. Although the easiest to define, predictive validity is possibly the most difficult to achieve. Predictive validity refers to whether we can predict an individual's performance and behaviours based on the results of their assessments. Naturally, the more isolated the assessment events are (as with terminal examinations and practical testing), the less predictive validity can be said to exist. Generally speaking, the more continuous the process the greater the predictive validity.

# Reliability

The reliability of an assessment is in some ways only a matter of degree. If for instance we devised a completely "reliable" assessment then a student would gain exactly the same result if they completed the assessment on more than one occasion. There are important factors outside the assessment strategy which will have a strong influence over this occurrence. The student's physical condition, mental state, environment, home circumstances, etc. will all affect their performance. Hence the reliability of an assessment is difficult to achieve. If however, a group of students of similar abilities and experiences undertake, a multiple choice question paper and achieve wildly differing results then it could be said with some certainty that this was an unreliable assessment. The use of pilot schemes to test the reliability of an assessment must involve large numbers of students in order to offset novel personal circumstances which may alter the results.

# Continuous assessment

The use of periodic assessment, as has been discussed, will at the very least, provide us with very little reliability and questionable validity in assessment of any type. It is known that reliability will increase the longer the assessment is carried on. It makes sense, therefore, to redesign assessment strategies into a continuous format which integrates both formative and summative assessments. Continuous assessment is a concept which embraces and integrates different assessment strategies into a unified approach and as such is arguably not an assessment method in its own right, but rather a philosophy of assessment. In other words it can be defined as "a planned series of progressively up-dated measurements of student achievement and progress" (ENB, 1986).

The use of continuous assessment in nurse education has been a feature of nursing curricula since 1988 and according to the ENB (1988) must meet certain criteria. Apart from the legal requirements with regard to the Nurses, Midwives, Health Visitors Approval Order No. 873 1983 (19(1)(c)) which each strategy has to meet, it is also necessary that such a strategy reflects a curriculum in which theory and practice are related.

If it is assumed that in the curricula, theory reflects practice and *vice versa*; it should, and indeed is, feasible within a framework of continuous assessment to devise separate assessment strategies for each. As far as dividing the curricula for assessment purposes is concerned, this is usually looked at in terms of "parts" which comprise smaller units. Each part should have a set of component assessments which maximise validity and reliability, incorporate formative and summative assessment and reflect "the acquisition of knowledge, skills, attitudes and competencies of differing complexity and application". (ENB, 1988).

# Profiles

Representing the data obtained from assessments, particularly if a continuous assessment strategy has been used, can present problems. In recent years, one way of overcoming this problem has been through the use of *profiles*. According to Frith and Macintosh (1984) "The term Profile is used to describe multidimensional methods of presenting information usually about individuals and their achievements, attributes or performances." The major differences between different profiles is not surprisingly their content and method of presentation but as Frith and Macintosh go on to point out, they should all have the following characteristics:

1. Lists of items such as skills, competencies, subjects and personal attributes.
2. Some way of indicating the level achieved.
3. A way of indicating what evidence supports the grades arrived at.

A profile is therefore a method of visually presenting information obtained through assessment either formatively or summatively and through a variety of strategies which may be mentor-, peer- or self-assessed. In its most basic form, a profile could just provide a list of marks obtained for various subjects throughout the curriculum as distinct from an overall mark. More commonly, however, the following profiles are used.

## Numerical rating scale (Figure 9.1)

On the positive side, this design of profile is easy to use, but the example given is open to wide interpretation. Therefore alongside such a scale, clear guidelines would need to be given as to the meaning of each skill and each level of achievement. Consequently, a tool such as this which on first inspection appears easy to design and use may, in the long run be neither. Its major uses would be where the skills being assessed were not open to interpretation (e.g. resuscitation training) rather than where they deal with more complicated behaviour.

---

**Topic: Communication**

Circle the number most appropriate:

1 = Needs further practice

2 = Adequate level achieved

3 = Shows aptitude

4 = Excellent level of practice

*Comments*

Listening skills:      1   2   3   4

Information giving:      1   2   3   4

Response to questions:   1   2   3   4

Conveying messages:    1   2   3   4

---

**Figure 9.1.** Numerical rating scale.

## Grid profile

The information contained on a grid profile gives more detail as to the different levels of competence which has been achieved and hence requires less subjective judgement. It may still, as with our example, be numerical in nature:

| Communication | 1 | 2 | 3 | 4 |
|---|---|---|---|---|
| Conveying messages | Conveys the basic meaning of message | | | Conveys messages effectively |

With these guidelines in mind, we now have to turn our attention towards the problem of how assessment will actually take place in the clinical setting and how the more theoretical components of assessment can be used in the clinical area.

## Assessment strategies in nursing

Nursing, like virtually any other profession, has two readily identifiable components (theory and practice) which, in the learning environment, should become increasingly more indivisible as the student progresses through the course. The dilemma has, for some years, been how to overcome the problem of having separate assessment strategies for each. The final written examination and the continuous assessment of both practice and course work should complement each other so as to overcome these difficulties. The reader must naturally reach their own conclusions as to whether this goal has been achieved for students in their area.

Refinements have occurred in the last decade as we have progressed from a system of having isolated and unique practical assessments to continuous assessment (ENB, 1987) and from central to devolved examination systems. These two policy changes have ensured that not only are national standards met but that they are also sensitive to local conditions and experiences. There is however, a certain degree of flexibility within guidelines issued which allow individual examination boards to develop their own formal assessments whilst ensuring that competencies are adequately assessed.

Taken that continuous assessment is the vehicle in which types of assessment must be placed and that further there must be a combination of formative and summative assessment, it now seems appropriate to examine some of the types of assessment which may be used.

## Methods of assessment

There are many ways of classifying types of assessment. They could, for instance be said to be student centred or teacher centred, but this may be misleading because some types may incorporate both, such as with projects. We have already discussed earlier Rowntree's classification and seen that most assessments are a combination of approaches. The ENB (1987) has stated that a continuous assessment format "may be of a form that takes into account the students' needs and preferences", but at the same time it must demonstrate that a predetermined level of competence has been reached. For the purposes of our discussion, therefore, no attempt has been made to categorise the types of assessment into one category or another as this is dependent on so many differing factors (e.g. the personality and teaching style of the teacher) that it would be misleading.

## Peer- and self-assessment

The concept that assessment can be carried out introspectively or with peers has gained momentum in recent years (e.g. Burnard, 1987). Its advantages are clear to see in as far as it tends to be less threatening to an individual to identify their own strengths and weaknesses either on their own or with their equals. The disadvantages are similarly immediately obvious, particularly in relation to its possibly threatening nature with regard to revealing weaknesses to a peer group. An outline of how peer- and self-assessment can be organised is given below (adapted from Burnard, 1987) and may serve as a foundation for setting up groups for this purpose.

1. Establish by consent a group of individuals who wish to be involved in this form of activity.
2. Establish confidentiality rules within the group in order that individuals will feel free to express themselves.
3. Set aside times for regular meetings and, if possible, give each meeting a function, e.g. to examine the rough drafts of a dissertation or project that everyone would have completed.
4. Each individual will have prepared not only their draft but will also have made notes about its strengths and weaknesses and perhaps even their thoughts for future work.
5. If common problems are found through informal discussions before the meetings, such as difficulty interpreting the criteria being used to assess the piece of work, then clarification should be sought from the relevant tutor.
6. At the meeting, each individual presents their work uninterrupted and with their own self-criticisms for a period of, e.g. 10 minutes.
7. Following this activity, the group then discusses the individual's work and comments before moving on to the next individual and repeating the process.

The inherent dangers will be largely overcome by each student having to present their work in turn although it has to be said that those students who the rest of the group consider as more advanced may present a threat to the others.

## Portfolios

One particular vehicle for assessment, the *portfolio*, can be identified as predominantly student centred, and largely self-assessed in a formative sense. A portfolio can be loosely described as a collection of varied materials such as journals which by definition will include the individual's reflections (see below), profiles, project work, results of peer- and self-assessments.

Portfolios could be said to form "a loose and untested constellation of innovative projects" (Glen and Hight, 1992). The content of a portfolio is quite naturally a possible consequence of self-direction and hence will be largely subjective and therefore divorced from the curriculum. In terms of its ideal applications, as Glen and Hight point out, it is well suited to the adult learner. In assessment terms, unless rigid direction and guidelines are given, its principal uses will be formative and will focus on the characteristics given above for formative assessments.

# Journals

The journal or diary as a method of self-assessment (Burnard, 1988) is seen as an integral part of the reflective process and hence enables students to complete at least a part of the learning cycle as described by Kolb (1984). As Burnard points out a journal or diary requires that entries are made on a weekly basis and could include the following, but may be adapted by the individual:

1. Problems encountered and the resolution of those problems.
2. Likes and dislikes of work experience.
3. New learning, including new references, skills, disorders, treatments, etc.
4. Application of learning to nursing.
5. Notes on self-development.
6. Other comments.

The use of journals for some students may be beneficial even in terms of a summative assessment (Scriven, 1967) in so far as individual criteria for the assessment of the journal may be worked out between the student and teacher. This would only fulfil some of the criteria for summative assessment, and if nomothetic and convergent aspects are to be assessed, then these have to be within broad areas of, for instance, referencing, writing style and other generalities which have little to do with the content. Some students, however, will not warm to the task and the journal may be of little use to them in any meaningful sense.

Formatively, the journal or diary is an immensely useful tool, considering as it does the progression from inexperience to experience, and it has the intrinsic value of being student centred; hence it provides a sensitive measurement of the individual's development.

Diaries or journals can on some courses be compulsory and by definition will be open to scrutiny if part of the assessment process is performed by anyone other than the person completing it. Its effectiveness as a truthful document and an accurate reflection of what is actually being felt and experienced must be called into question. To overcome this problem to some extent, a part of the journal needs to be identified as private and access restricted to the student.

The student's personal accounts of satisfying/unsatisfying experiences used in this case as part of a journal, can form part of a needs-assessment strategy (MacDonald and Grogin, 1991; Banfield, 1990). The journal can be used in this context to form a basis with which to identify the future learning needs of the student by analysing the gap between what is actually known and what needs to be known. Using it in this way, the use of contracts (see below) is arguably more relevant.

# Case studies

Many of us who have taught students in the clinical area will be familiar (though perhaps not by name) with a strategy of teaching and assessment known as case studies. Traditionally descriptive case studies (care studies) have been used as a form of project work where the student will identify a patient or client and write about their problems and the care given. This may be of benefit for some students in terms of being able to integrate theory into practice. In education terms, case studies may have a much wider use and have almost certainly been encountered by most of us at some time or another. In this second context, a case study is a problem-solving and analysis exercise based on real or simulated scenarios and may be completed by an individual or a group.

Case studies may take several forms and may be designed to fit any level from, e.g. basic care to fairly complex management situations. Broadly speaking, the most applicable case studies to use in the clinical area are as follows.

## Critical incidence case study

A series of incidents leading up to and including the penultimate event of a situation are described. The task of the student is to identify what they need to find out in order to complete the picture and to define the full circumstances, e.g.

Mr Smith is admitted to the surgical unit for routine repair of hernia. He arrives at 0830 h with his wife, who departs a few minutes later. Upon his first contact with you, he appears nervous and agitated. He is due to go to theatre at 1000 h and despite the data obtained at admission not identifying any obvious problems regarding his physical well-being, you are worried that either he is not psychologically prepared for surgery or that something else is causing him concern.

What additional information would you require in order to complete a more comprehensive assessment of Mr Smith's psychological state and how would you go about obtaining it?

## Next-stage case study

With this case study, a series of events is revealed to the student and he/she are required to identify what is most likely to happen next. This will require a high degree of analysis and the ability to pull together information, e.g.

Mr Jones moved in with his daughter and family largely because, although fit, he was mentally unable to care for himself at home. His behaviour had always been described as strange by relatives and he had been living alone in squalid conditions since the death of his wife 10 years earlier. He was largely cared for by his daughter and her husband but this took the form of mental support and physical chores. The relationship between Mr Jones and the rest of the family, including three children, was not close. Five years ago Mr Jones developed a vascular disorder which led to gangrene for which he persistently refused the advised surgical treatment. He has been visited daily for the last five years by the community nursing team for the dressing to be changed.

Within the last year, both the son-in-law and daughter have visited the GP because they maintain that Mr Jones's mental state has deteriorated considerably. So far, social services, psychiatrist and community psychiatric nurse have all visited and identified that there is a problem, but stated that there is nothing they can do. It is obvious that all concerned in the family are under considerable pressure.

Given the above facts, what could be the possible consequences to this situation?

## The live case study

As distinct from the next-stage case study, the live case study asks what should be done next rather than what will happen next. Taking the above example, it is easy to see that a different outcome to the scenario can be brought about by asking the question:

In the above situation what actions would you take to prevent this situation deteriorating further?

The use of case studies in the ways mentioned above is a common feature of many written examinations but they can be used very effectively in the clinical situation as an impromptu or planned method of assessing the student's ability to analyse, comprehend and, to an extent, deal with various situations.

## Skills of the assessor

The interviews that take place between the student and mentor during and at the end of an experience should be seen as an important part of the education process. Students need to have regular discussions about their progress during an experience in order to make any changes to their practice that are required.

This process is commonly seen as one person making a judgement on the performance of another. This is fine when the student has performed well in the view of the teacher/mentor, but when placed in the position of having to be critical, many people find the process uncomfortable or even threatening. The reason for this is that they may feel that they are in the position of making a unilateral decision about the performance of the student, that the responsibility is all theirs, that these decisions may affect the whole future of that student and, in some instances, could lead to the end of the student's course. This commonly leads to the teacher/mentor not making a reasoned decision at all but marking the student as average.

By applying the concepts outlined in this chapter, it will be seen that the decision-making process is a shared one made by the student, the mentor, other trained staff who have worked with the student, the ward sister, the ward teacher, the student's course teacher and, in some instances, the course director. When viewed in this light, the decisions that have to be made become much easier and of course much more balanced.

The first step in this process is to look at the structure of the interviews that are to take place. Keeping in mind that this is an important part of the student's education process, i.e. the need to develop "self-appraisal skills", we need to consider that all students are individuals and accept that one structure may not be suitable for all of them.

## Summary

The subject of assessment involves factors which relate to how an individual learns, how an individual puts their learning into practice and even the psychological and logistical factors involved in attempting to ascertain how much learning has taken place.

The trend away from periodic practice-based assessments to continuous assessment to some extent reflects the complexities both of the learning process and of the nature of nursing itself.

Broadly speaking, formative assessment refers to the process of ascertaining a student's progress during a course of study or experience in, usually, an informal way.

Summative assessment on the other hand involves the assessing of learning which has taken place and hopefully applied to practice and is most obviously typified by a final examination.

Validity can be said to be "an examination of the approximate truth or falsity of the propositions" (Cook and Campbell, 1979). Put more simply it is "a measure of the truth or accuracy of a claim" (Burns and Grove, 1987).

Continuous assessment can be defined as "a planned series of progressively up-dated measurements of student achievement and progress" (ENB, 1986).

A profile is a method of visually presenting information obtained through assessment either formatively or summatively and through a variety of strategies.

Assessment is a learning opportunity and can form a useful basis for further development.

# Related activities

## Activity 1

With reference to a course that you help to facilitate, identify the following:

1. The formative and summative components of the assessment strategy.
2. The assessment strategies employed.

## Activity 2

With reference to the assessment strategy of the course that you have investigated, write short notes on how predictive validity is assured with the strategies that are employed.

# References

Banfield, V., Brooks, E., Brown, J. *et al.* (1990) A strategy to identify the learning needs of staff nurses. *Journal of Continuing Education in Nursing*, **21**(5), 209–211.

Burnard, P. (1987) Self and peer assessment. *Senior Nurse*, **6**(5), 16–17.

Burnard, P. (1988) Journal as an assessment and evaluation tool in nurse education ... journal or diary. *Nurse Education Today*, **8**(2), 105–107.

Burns, N. and Grove, S. (1987) *The Practice of Nursing Research Conduct Critique and Utilisation*. Philadelphia: W.B. Saunders.

Cook, T.D. and Campbell, D.T. (1979) *Quasi experimentation: design and analysis for field settings*. Chicago: Rand McNally College Publishing. (In N. Burns and S. Grove *The Practice of Nursing Research Conduct Critique and Utilisation*. Philadelphia: W.B. Saunders.)

ENB (1986) Devolved final written examinations. (1986 /30/ ERDB.)

ENB (1987) Devolved continuous assessment for theory in first level nursing courses.

ENB (1988) Devolved continuous assessment.

Frith, D.S. and Macintosh, H.G. (1984) *A Teacher's Guide to Self-assessment*. Cheltenham: Stanley Thornes.

Glen, S. and Hight, N. (1992) Portfolios: an "affective" assessment strategy? *Nurse Education Today*, **12**(6), 416–423.

Kilty, J. (1977) Self and peer assessment and peer audit human potential resource project. University of Surrey, Guilford.

Kolb (1984) *Experiential Learning: Experience as a Source of Learning and Development*. Englewood Cliffs, Prentice Hall.

MacDonald, R. and Grogin, E.R. (1991) Personal accounts of satisfying and unsatisfying nursing experiences as a needs assessment strategy. *Journal of Continuing Education in Nursing*, **22**(1), 11–15.

Rowntree, D. (1977) *Assessing Students: How Shall We Know Them*. London: Harper and Row.

Scriven, M. (1967) The methodology of education. In R.O. Tyler, R.M. Gagne and M. Scriven (eds) *Perspective of Curriculum Evaluation*. AERA Monograph Series on Curriculum Evaluation No. 1. Chicago: Rand McNally.

# chapter ten

# Education resources

## Introduction

When considering education resources, it is easy to suppose that these are most applicable to the classroom situation and subsequently to build any discussion around this area alone. The traditional meaning of "education resources" has perhaps, in the past, centred on library facilities, whiteboards, classroom arrangements, etc. The use of the term "education resources" in the clinical environment is no less important, and if we consider the learning environment as a combination of both formal college-based education and clinical experience, then these should be considered together. The emphasis in this chapter, however, is naturally biased towards the clinical environment and the resources that can be most effectively utilised there.

Reinforcement of information visually or by other means will go some way to ensuring that such information is more readily integrated by the student; further, the availability of resources in the clinical area will serve to enhance the student's experience in the more immediate situation and hence add relevance to the subject. Conversely, visual aids such as videos without the back-up of the preceptor may prove to be ineffective (Baldwin *et al.*, 1991). Probably the best place to start before we examine how to produce audio-visual aids is to examine the possibility of setting up an education resource area in the clinical environment which can be utilised by both students and trained staff.

## Building an education resources area

The resources that any clinical area may have extend far beyond just journals and textbooks. The whole subject of audio-visual aids is covered elsewhere in the next section, but for the purposes of our discussion here, a short list of possible resources is given. It will be noticed that a significant resource area can be developed for relatively little cost, and it is advisable to have a specific area set aside for such resources, and most certainly to have a named person responsible for it, perhaps on a rota basis.

1. *Journals.* Collected either from individuals who order particular journals on a regular basis, or by ward/unit subscriptions. Some discussion with staff about the selection of these journals is appropriate in order to ensure their most effective use.
2. *Abstracts.* Health Service Abstracts and especially Nursing Research Abstracts which are available from the Department of Health for a small annual fee can be extremely useful (see Chapter five).
3. *Textbooks.* Find out whether there is a fund from which the finance for textbooks can be provided. Hoarding of out-of-date and therefore, almost certainly irrelevant texts should be avoided.
4. *References.* There are several ways to build up a collection of relevant references. One

possible method is for a member of staff to be delegated each month to scan the appropriate journals and to record a brief summary of each one which could then form the basis of a reference section.

5. *Product information*. Manufacturers' information about their products which are being used in the clinical area is very important. Drugs, appliances and equipment will all have information relating to their use, as well as (in many cases) published research which justifies its use. All this information could be held centrally in a resource area.

6. *External agencies*. Information from national organisations self-help groups, and even relevant government agencies which may be applicable to the client group.

7. *Health education literature*. This resource is readily available, usually free of charge and highly recommended.

8. *Projects and local research*. These may have been carried out by members of staff as part of a course, or by past students or medical staff.

9. *Department information*. Detailing the services offered by other departments in the hospital.

10. *Contact Names*. Staff throughout the unit (or indeed outside) who are useful aids to the student (e.g. environmental health, dietician).

The education resource area should not remain the province of students on placements but should also cater for professional updating of staff undergoing specialist courses, management innovations as well as more general updating, gained from information found in journals, whether nursing or specialities allied to it (medicine, etc.). Links with other resource areas are immensely useful as this will not only increase the resources available to the individual but will also serve as a forum for sharing ideas about how to maintain and further develop such an area. One method which may be utilised effectively is the use of a journal club, either solely for that particular area or shared with other areas. With this club, a member, or members, of staff may be delegated on a monthly basis to review the literature concerning their speciality and other professionally relevant material and to bring it to the attention of their colleagues, perhaps during ward meetings.

# What audio-visual aids can do

Aside from the education resource area which can be considered as a visual aid in its own right, other audio-visual aids can be utilised effectively in the clinical environment. For instance, the use of an overhead projector is often well advised for certain teaching sessions. All that is required for most projection equipment is a power point and a blank wall, rather than using expensive screens.

Audio-visual aids are effective for:

1. *Developing additional communication channels*. Although the use of the voice is the most obvious audio aid, it is not necessarily the most effective and a variety of communication modes is advisable to maintain interest and attention.

2. *Forming connections between theory and practice*. Subjects such as physiology can obviously be enhanced using audio-visual aids, but also subjects where there are relationships between different components of the same subject may also be improved (e.g. looking at support services in the community and how they relate to the individual's discharge from hospital).

3. *Clarifying information*. Some concepts are difficult to explain without the use of an

additional channel of communication. Prostheses, anatomical models, etc., may serve to help the individual fully understand, e.g. the process and implications of surgery.

4. *Consolidation.* There are times when the information which has been presented or has been gained through experience needs to be summarised or presented in a different way in order for the individual to see it in context.

# Audio-visual aids commonly used

1. Overhead projector (OHP).
2. Flipchart.
3. Whiteboard.
4. Slides.
5. Videos.
6. Posters.

For the use of overhead projector, flipchart and whiteboard certain factors need to be borne in mind. Firstly, it does not take an artist to produce an effective visual aid but rather someone who has thought about their visual aid carefully and has taken a little time over its production. Secondly, and this cannot be emphasised strongly enough: don't become an aid for your visual aids!

Thirdly, some visual aids, particularly those which have been badly produced, may actually be detrimental to the session. Fourthly, some visual aids may be extremely artistic and very complex but they have very little value and may either serve to confuse or may overload the student with information.

Not everyone is especially good at producing visual aids but with the following criteria, the likelihood of being effective will be increased:

1. **Work** – it should work for the session being given.
2. **Appropriate** – in terms of level, content and context.
3. **Relevant** – to the subject and student(s).
4. **Timing** – should fit in at an appropriate juncture.
5. **Simple** – should be direct and to the point.

6. **Nominal cost** – should not be disproportionate to teaching value.

7. **Appealing** – maintains attention and may use novelty.
8. **Likelihood of success** – must be useful to the students.
9. **Limiting** – should apply to a small section of the session.

"WARTS N ALL" can be applied to any visual aid and can act as a checklist when preparing material. It is a common mistake for those new to teaching to spend a disproportionate amount of time preparing visual aids only to find that they are of little or no use.

One of the most important skills involved in producing visual aids is the ability to make writing legible, and hence a little time needs to be spent in examining this subject.

# Lettering

1. It is a good idea to consider which colours will be used to ensure clear visibility and which

colours go together to maximise their effect. The choice of colours will depend upon whether students are close to the screen or in a larger classroom.

Colours most visible close-up: black and ivory; green and ivory; black and orange; green and white.
Colours most visible from a distance: black and yellow; black and white; red and white; green and white.

When using an overhead projector (OHP), the screen can be classed as ivory and it should be remembered that it is not necessary to stick to only one colour per acetate but that it can be made more effective using a combination of colours. When presenting diagrams, the choice of colour is less crucial in relation to visibility but is nevertheless just as relevant when trying to emphasise a particular aspect (e.g. blood flow through the heart). It should be remembered that the use of colour can be rather overdone with lettering and should be restricted to two or three at most.

2. Freehand lettering has more character but if your handwriting is illegible on paper it will be far worse on an acetate. It may be better to consider the use of stencils or a lettering system. When writing on a flipchart or whiteboard, legibility can be increased by either writing the information in advance or at least planning what is to be written instead of leaving it until the session.
3. All written information should be clear, concise and spelt correctly.
4. When preparing an acetate, use lined paper underneath to ensure correct spacing, lettering size and tidiness.
5. In order to improve the tidiness of an acetate, a border may be drawn around the inside approximately half an inch from the edge.
6. With the above qualifications in mind, experiment with different lettering sizes and cases.
7. Decide how you wish to emphasise key words and keep it consistent.
8. Always test the legibility by viewing the image from the position where the students will be sitting.
9. Decide whether to use permanent or water-soluble pens; remember that the soluble pens will rub off when handled.

## Use of the overhead projector

1. Check screen is angled correctly to avoid "keystoning".
2. Ensure that the whole group can see the image; screen should be about six feet above the ground, and OHP positioned correctly, e.g. centre or corner position.
3. Ensure each acetate is focused correctly. (Check with the group to make sure those at the back can see.)
4. Do not stand in front of the image.
5. Point to the acetate rather than the screen to highlight points.
6. Allow enough time for the message to be understood and questions to be asked.
7. Turn OHP off when not in use.

## Use of the whiteboard

1. Ensure your handwriting is clear. A common error is to write too quickly when teaching – take your time!

2. Diagrams should be clear and understandable. (You may like to prepare these before your presentation.)
3. Avoid standing with your back to the group for too long.
4. Avoid talking while you are writing; this will distance you from the group and makes for poor communication.
5. When writing suggestions from the group, use their exact words; this helps to involve the group and encourages participation.

## Use of slides

Although it is not common to use slides in the clinical area, it is sometimes the case that a member of staff has a particularly useful set of slides which can illustrate a concept such as an operative procedure.

1. Make sure that you understand how to use the equipment. (Practise on your own if necessary.)
2. Plan carefully when the slides will be used during your session (avoid the use of slides, or any other medium, alone). Variety helps to keep the group's attention.
3. Ensure that your slides are in the right order, the right way round and in focus before the session.
4. Simply turning off the lights should be enough to make the image clear, so avoid darkening the room if possible. It is difficult to concentrate in the dark and this reduces group participation.

## Use of videos

Interactive videos can be very useful to enhance learning in a specific area. Take care to avoid the use of pre-recorded TV programmes which may infringe the copyright laws. As mentioned earlier, visual aids without the opportunity for discussion are often ineffective.

## Use of posters

The use of posters as an educational aid is known to us all within the realms of health education, although their usage in professional education can be considerable if used correctly. Naturally a poster can be designed in a variety of ways, but there are certain guidelines which can facilitate their effectiveness.

### Poster size

It has been suggested that the optimum size for a poster is about $32 \times 40$ inches (Seigal, 1992), although this will naturally depend on the space available. Materials should be carefully chosen, with their usage firmly in mind. If the poster is to be used over a long period of time, for instance, a thicker board will be required, otherwise it will have to be replaced after a short period.

## *Purpose*

If the poster is designed to help the student to complement existing preset learning outcomes, then these should be identified on the poster. If the purpose is for general updating, such as will be used for cardiopulmonary resuscitation, then previous policies that it is intended to replace should be included. If conveying a policy or procedure, then the complete document from which it is derived should be available.

## *Location*

If the poster is to bring the attention of staff to, for instance, policy changes, then naturally these should be placed in an area of "high traffic", i.e. where staff will have to pass it several times a day (or ideally come face-to-face with it!).

Otherwise, the general information given earlier on the preparation of visual aids is applicable ("WARTS N ALL").

## The patient/relative as a visual aid

Most obviously, the most effective visual aids of all in the clinical area, are the individuals upon which teaching is centred, namely the patients and relatives. Naturally, the individuals concerned need to be aware of any teaching process that is going on and need to have given their consent for this to happen. Having done so, the patient may provide valuable information in terms of verbal reporting of problems, visual aspects such as wound healing, rehabilitation, in fact any aspect of the patient's day-to-day care.

Note that patients should not be used to practice on unless the "service" is required by them, e.g. taking/recording of blood pressure.

One consequence of using the patient/relative as an audio-visual aid is the implication that emotional aspects of treatment may be explored. Talking to individuals about their feelings on dying for instance may provide vast amounts of useful information, but if handled badly may disrupt the individual's coping mechanisms. Much more useful information can be gleaned by normal social interaction and a building of relationships over a period of time. It is of course likely that there may be individuals who have dealt with their situation so well that they wish to impart their experiences and knowledge to others. This is particularly the case when talking to some carers in the home situation whose relatives have come into hospital for further investigations or respite care. It should be remembered that it is often the carer at home who can offer more insight into the day-to-day management of care than can the trained professional.

## Conclusions

The use of audio-visual aids in the clinical area is a vital component of the learning environment. The education resource area, although vital, should not be considered in isolation from other areas but rather as a part of a large resource available to individuals. This must invariably include college facilities and resources, particularly libraries, but also areas where students will be directed to use aids which are not available in the clinical area (such as computer-assisted learning). It is a mistake to assume that an effective resource area needs to be an expensive one. The key to success appears to be the communication between staff in different areas rather than the isolation of individual areas with little outside interaction.

# Summary

The resources that any clinical area may have extend far beyond just journals and textbooks.

The education resource area should not remain the province of students on placements but should also cater for professional updating of staff undergoing specialist courses.

Links with other resource areas are immensely useful as this will not only increase the resources available to the individual but will also serve as a forum for sharing ideas about how to maintain and further develop such an area.

Audio-visual aids are effective for:

1. Developing additional communication channels.
2. Forming connections between theory and practice
3. Clarifying information
4. Consolidation

The following should be considered when preparing visual aids:

1. **Work** – it should work for the session being given.
2. **Appropriate** – in terms of level, content and context.
3. **Relevant** – to the subject and student(s).
4. **Timing** – should fit in at an appropriate juncture.
5. **Simple** – should be direct and to the point.
6. **Nominal cost** – should not be disproportionate to teaching value.
7. **Appealing** – maintains attention and may use novelty.
8. **Likelihood of success** – must be useful to the students.
9. **Limiting** – Should apply to a small section of the session.

Most obviously, the most effective visual aids of all in the clinical area, are the individuals upon which teaching is centred, namely the patients and relatives.

# Related activities

## Activity 1. Developing clinical education resources

1. Make a list of the education resources available in your clinical area.
2. What are the publication dates of any texts and have there been any subsequent editions? (Can be found in individual publisher's catalogues or Meditec. See Appendix two.)
3. Which method is used to enable individuals to find the information available? (index, library cards, etc.)
4. Is there a method of recording which resources are used most frequently?
5. Identify another area similar to your own and compare the above results with theirs.
6. Write a short report for your ward manager detailing the resources which need to be purchased/updated.

If, whilst carrying out this activity, it is found that the resources are used very little then some time needs to be spent in ascertaining why this is the case. It may be that the area is inacessible, i.e. in an office or that the material is not relevant or up-to-date.

## Activity 2. Production of a visual aid

1. Select a teaching/learning experience in your clinical area.
2. Produce, using the above guidelines, either an overhead projector transparency or poster to be used in the session.
3. Write a short (200 words) rationale explaining your choice of visual aid.
4. Record how long it took to prepare it.
5. Evaluate its effectiveness after the session.

# References

Baldwin, D., Hill, P. and Hanson, G., (1991) Performance of psychomotor skills: a comparison of two teaching strategies. *Journal of Nursing Education*, **30**(8), 367–370.

Seigal, H. (1992) Innovative approaches to inservice education. *The Journal of Continuing Education in Nursing*, **22**(4), 147–151.

# chapter eleven

# Participation in curriculum planning

## Introduction

Participation in curriculum planning groups (sometimes called Course Scheme Development Groups) is now a feature of the professional nurse's life and indeed is the requirement of the National Boards (e.g. ENB, 1987). It is a common mistake to assume that participating in such a group merely means deciding upon which topics are to be covered in the course over a given amount of time. This is not surprising as curriculum planning by its very nature is governed by professional knowledge, education expertise and copious national syllabi, as well as numerous internal organisational factors.

The individual who is asked to participate in the curriculum planning group should ideally not only have a good idea about what is to be achieved in terms of content, but also should have a knowledge of the curriculum models being used, the teaching strategies being utilised and perhaps most importantly of all, an understanding through participation of the philosophy of the planning team towards the education of the individual.

As with most other areas of education, curriculum planning encompasses a wide scope of concepts, few of which will be utilised in an unadapted form. This is by no means a criticism of the systems which are utilised, but nevertheless, cautionary observation should be made before we begin our discussion. Debates regarding the nature of teaching are a frequent occurrence in curriculum planning groups, in particular within the realms of behavioural and more process-based approaches. The arguments against behavioural objectives, for instance, have been voiced loudly by authors such as Stenhouse (1975) but, on the other hand, they have been widely adopted by many. Debates such as this cannot be seen in isolation from a national syllabus and the conditions which are set down by governing bodies. It is not unreasonable to assume that there may be a difference between what the curriculum planning group sets out and what is actually carried out in practice, although of course, with appropriate planning and representation, this should not occur.

It can be seen that the curriculum planning process is most certainly not an activity confined to one small group but rather it is a process which must include all those involved in the learning process, and this must have implications for in-service and post-basic education as well as, most obviously, the links between the college and the clinical area. If discord occurs, for whatever reason, the hard work put in by those involved in curriculum planning may be wasted.

# Developments in nurse education

The enormous changes that have occurred in nurse education in particular since 1989 (with the advent of Project 2000), have brought with them not only educational innovations, but also in terms of organisational changes. Drastic though these changes have been, the majority of them have been recommended (to some extent at least) for over twenty years in various reports. Briggs (1972), to name only one report has recommended dramatic changes within the system.

Eventually, after extensive consultation, the UKCC presented its guidelines and criteria for Project 2000 to the profession, and for the purposes of our discussion on curriculum development, some of the major points are outlined below (adapted from ENB, 1989).

1. All pre-registration courses should be taught to Diploma level as a minimum standard.
2. Nurse education institutions must have a collaborative link with Higher Education institutions (being a standard higher than GCE "A" Level and examinations for the national certificate or National Diploma or the Business and Technical Education Council).
3. Courses should be conjointly validated between the Higher Education Institution and the National Boards to ensure the correct academic standard. This process is somewhat less cumbersome than on first appearance, as many nurse education institutions have actually become integrated into universities.
4. All students entering pre-registration courses must complete a common foundation course comprising 2300 curricular hours (18 months). The same allocation of hours applies to each of the four branch programmes making a total of 4600 hours (three years).
5. Out of the 4600 total curricular hours, 50% should be designated for learning within practice setting.
6. A total of no more than 20% of the course (six months) will be designated as a rostered contribution to nursing service.
7. The rostered service must be educationally led, usually in the third year of the course within a team led by an appropriately qualified first level nurse.

Although the reader is naturally directed to the original document, the above brief outline should give some idea as to the direction that the planning of practical-based education should go. The UKCC is also at pains to point out that experience should be gained in a wide variety of settings and that student choice is an important consideration, and further that appropriate support must be provided. Perhaps one observation that should be made at this point is that this form of nurse education, whilst firmly establishing an academic basis, is by no means a solely classroom-based system and that the practice component is crucial to the development of the individual student.

# Preparing to participate in a curriculum development group

The amount of information governing the development of a new curriculum can be immensely bewildering. It is very easy to become a sleeping partner in the curriculum planning process if the appropriate documentation and facts have not been given to the participants beforehand. This of course should not happen in an efficient curriculum planning group. It is difficult to conceive that everyone involved in the planning process has a complete and in-depth knowledge of every document, both internal and external, which will govern its development, and it is highly desirable to raise questions to the appropriate personnel if you are not sure as to the relevance and nature of some of the information you have been given. Below is a brief checklist which may be utilised when asked to participate in a curriculum planning group:

1. Current regulations and guidelines for the approval of courses (national and local) e.g. Nurses, Midwives and Health Visitors Act (1989) Rule 18A (see Appendix Four).
2. Relevant National Board information pertaining to the course.
3. Existing curriculum for course being planned (if in existence).
4. College philosophy.
5. Documents pertaining to assessment strategy (both local and national).
6. Minutes and other information from previous meetings (if joining after the inaugural meeting).
7. Any information pertaining to anticipated changes within the clinical area that may affect the experience offered.
8. Access to clinical audit documents of areas to be used as clinical placements.
9. Information regarding college structure and monitoring systems, e.g. quality control.
10. List of dates of planning meetings.

It is not a good idea to participate in such a group without any preparation and this may include:

1. Scanning the above material and perhaps making short notes on the point you wish to be clarified.
2. Discussing with colleagues items on the agenda that they feel are important.
3. Discussing with appropriate nurse teacher any queries that you have.

Each member of the curriculum planning group has by virtue of their experience useful contributions to make. The plethora of information generated for and by a curriculum planning group can be off-putting, although this should not be the case and there will be many experienced staff to provide support if necessary. At this juncture it is appropriate to examine an actual (abridged) curriculum/course management team's terms of reference.

*Composition of Course and Course Scheme Committees*
As a minimum, course and course scheme committees must include:

1. A course leader or course scheme director (chair).
2. Chairs of appropriate sub-committees.
3. Staff representatives from each major contributing element of the course or course scheme.
4. A representative sample of students.
5. External representatives and advisors as appropriate.
6. Resource managers as appropriate.

*Terms of Reference of Course Schemes and Course Scheme Committees*

The course or course scheme committee shall be responsible to the Senate of the University (through the Academic Board of the Regional College at which the student is enrolled) for the smooth running of the course or the course scheme, its academic quality and for the academic welfare of the students.
  Specifically, the committee shall be responsible for the following:

1. Achievement of course/course schemes outcomes.
2. Implementation of the aims and objective of the course/course scheme and oversight of the continuing appropriateness of the content.
3. Oversight of the operation of any sub-committee reporting to it.
4. Implementation and review of course/course scheme policy.
5. Maintenance of academic standards including monitoring and evaluation of course/course scheme.
6. Agreement of a periodic report on the course/course scheme according to the requirements of the Universities Senate.
7. Preparation of the information required for the renewal of approval or review of the course/course scheme or its constituent elements at appropriate intervals.

8. Nomination of proposed external assessors for onward transmission to the Senate or appropriate sub-committee.
9. Making of recommendations to the University or Regional College Executive on matters relating to the effective organisation and administration of the course/course scheme including resources.

(Reproduced by kind permission of Anglia Polytechnic University.)

# The curriculum planning process

Although there is diversity in how the curriculum planning process should proceed, it is nevertheless useful to consider a procedure which can dictate how the team progresses.

By necessity, the curriculum development is largely governed by the guidelines produced regarding the approvals process, as well as the course development regulations and guidelines. The needs of the community in terms of the scope and volume of care provided is important not only because of future staffing requirements but also when considering the effectiveness of the learning environment. There are, however, other factors involved in the process that have to be decided by the curriculum planning team, and first of these is the development of a course philosophy.

# The course philosophy/ideology

The course philosophy is developed in line with the philosophy of the college which will normally govern the general conduct of courses, the educational climate and even relationships between students, educationists and managers. The term philosophy can be argued by purists as sometimes being inappropriate, although in the context of being a commentary or system of theories on the nature of the education process, it is entirely appropriate. Conversely, the term ideology, which is a collection of beliefs of a group, more accurately reflects the deliberations of a curriculum planning team.

The development of a curriculum ideology must not only be a compilation of the ideas of the whole curriculum team, but should also reflect, through team members, the ideas and beliefs of those whom they represent. Failure to take account of the wider perspective of views will inevitably lead to an artifical ideology which has no bearing on reality. Further, lack of consultation will lead to lack of ownership on the part of those expected to implement it.

# Diagnosis of needs: developing curriculum models

Developing a curriculum model around which a more detailed curricular content can be organised is, on the surface, a relatively straightforward exercise. Curriculum teams will vary considerably in how they arrive at such a model, but nevertheless, whether formally or informally, the process is carried out in more than one stage. Naturally the determining factors that dictate the development of a model or the adoption of an existing one must be considered, and these can be said to fall broadly into the following categories:

1. The ideology of the college.
2. The ideology of the course.

3. The outline curriculum produced by the awarding body.
4. Local conditions and experiences available.

## The nature of nursing

One of the most crucial decisions to be made is the nature of nursing itself and the factors which influence the care that we give. The participation of practitioners involved in day-to-day care is crucial to this process if it is to be successful. It may be the case that the adoption and modification of an existing model of nursing (e.g. Orem, 1985; Peplau, 1952), may accurately reflect the beliefs of the group although with multi-branch education programmes in mind, this may be impossible. It seems far more likely that a more holistic view will be taken regarding the nature of nursing and that this may take the form of the outline shown in Figure 11.1.

## The nature of education – the process *vs* product debate

In recent years, much attention has been paid to the arguments which either advocate or refute a behaviourist approach to education. More specifically, concerns have been expressed regarding the nature of education in terms of whether it is viewed as a standard and predictable end product or whether the process of education should take prominence. A product-based curriculum relies heavily on behavioural objectives which by their very nature attempt to predict exactly what a student will have learned following an educational experience or course of study. Stenhouse (1975) encapsulates the process-based argument succinctly when he states that "... skills are probably susceptible to treatment through the objective model, which encounters its greatest problems in areas of knowledge".

The system of *behavioural objectives*, which were a familiar component of most nursing curricula, was based substantially on the work of Bloom (1956) and gained prominence in the 1960s and 70s. It had its uses particularly in the realms of skills training where the outcome of learning was directly observable and, to a large extent, predictable. Behavioural objectives, more specifically instructional objectives, attempt to dictate exactly what behaviours should

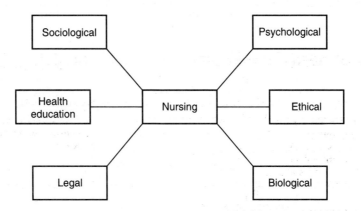

**Figure 11.1.** The nature of nursing.

result from a learning experience. An example of a behavioural objective would be:

At the end of the session the student will be able to list six signs and symptoms of congestive cardiac failure.

Although easy to evaluate (either they have or have not formed a list) the relevance of such instructional objectives has to be questioned both in terms of cognitive functioning and how the individual deals with the information they are presented with. As mentioned earlier, their application appears to be more relevant to skills training than to an education system which is attempting to produce a knowledgeable doer. Their demise in nurse education and the shift towards a process-based model is now becoming a common feature in curricular design (Rush *et al.*, 1991) and reflects a more "humanistic" approach to nurse education. By virtue of the fact that an objective-based product model is associated with a more mechanised form of training, it comes as no surprise that a shift over to a process model reflects a transition from nurse "training" to nurse "education" (Darbyshire, 1991).

The process model in its purest form concentrates on the education experience rather than a predictable education outcome and, not surprisingly, relies heavily on the individual learner as the central focus. The precise result of education is not known as the individual will undergo experiences and interpret learning encounters in a unique way. The increasing use of *learning outcomes*, as distinct from behavioural objectives, has become a common feature of nursing curricula.

Precise definitions of a learning outcome are sadly lacking in the literature, and for the purposes of our discussion the definitions offered by Stenhouse to what he termed "expressive objectives" would appear to be compatible with what is now known as learning outcomes. An expressive objective does not specify behaviours that students will be expected to attain following an experience or encounter, rather it identifies situations in which the individual will participate and serves as a theme around which skills and understandings can be brought to bear in an individual way (Stenhouse, 1975).

An example of an expressive objective/learning outcome would be:

To examine and appraise the nursing intervention required by a patient with a cardiovascular disorder.

It has to be said that as desirable as this model is, it is not entirely compatible with any system of education which incorporates a standardised final examination, as presently exists in

**Table 11.1.** Advantages/disadvantages of product (behaviourist) approach

| Advantages | Disadvantages |
| --- | --- |
| 1. Provides clear guidelines for students. | 1. Inhibits individuality in learning. |
| 2. Makes lesson planning easier. | 2. Does not take account of the cognitive |
| 3. Facilitates use of terminal examination. | processes involved. |
| 4. Easier to plan for experiences. | 3. Restricts the scope of learning by setting |
| 5. Comparison of student achievements is possible | specific terminal objectives. |
| 6. Effective in skills training. | 4. Ineffective in knowledge acquisition. |
| 7. Economical in terms of time. | 5. Restricts enquiry and analysis. |
| 8. Outcomes are measurable. | 6. Individual unique achievements difficult to |
| 9. Makes the comparison of different courses possible. | assess. |
| 10. Popular with students. | 7. Ignores the learning experience as valuable in itself. |
| | 8. Teacher directed. |

**Table 11.2.**    Advantages/disadvantages of process (humanistic) approach

| Advantages | Disadvantages |
| --- | --- |
| 1. Takes account the individual learning needs. | 1. May be very time consuming. |
| 2. Student centred. | 2. Teacher loses control of the learning experience. |
| 3. Values the process rather than the outcome of education. | 3. Difficult to maintain a national standard. |
| 4. Varying levels of students can be facilitated. | 4. May be too unstructured for some students. |
| 5. Students can work at their own pace. | 5. Uneconomic. |
| 6. Learning experiences are more meaningful and therefore more complete. | 6. Impossible to compare students. |
| 7. Encourages growth towards self-actualisation. | 7. Incompatible with a final examination. |
| 8. Increases self-esteem by not comparing with others. | 8. Does not assist the poor teacher! |
| 9. Does not depend on a terminal examination to judge prior learning. | 9. Difficult to plan. |
| | 10. Difficult to assess objectively. |
| | 11. Unpopular with some students. |

nursing. As Stenhouse points out,

... if the examination is a by-product, there is an implication that the quality the student shows in it must be an under-estimate of his real quality (Stenhouse, 1975).

It would be wrong to reject totally either the process-based or product-based system out of hand, each has its advantages and disadvantages (Tables 11.1 and 11.2).

The shift towards a process approach appears to be gaining momentum (Crotty, 1993) and this in many ways has to be seen as desirable in as much as it encourages the individual to reach their potential. To view either approach as a unique distinct entity, could be to ignore the realities of an education system which both encourages analysis and works to a national standard. Perhaps a more realistic way of viewing the approaches is to consider them as opposite ends of a continuum with a greater or lesser degree of each incorporated into nursing curricula. By virtue of having to attain competencies and by undertaking a standardised system of assessments, at least some part of the curriculum may be said to be product-based in nature.

# The curriculum model

Like any other planning exercise, course planning needs a framework around which its development will proceed. There are, however, factors involved in choosing a curriculum model which must be considered. The very phrase "choosing a curriculum model", is in itself misleading. In planning a curriculum three major factors have to be dealt with, each of which may have a separate model:

1. The course content.
2. Organisation of course material.
3. Learning strategies to be used for the course.

## The course content

The content, in broad terms, needs to be examined. The outlining syllabus provided by the awarding authority (National Boards) serve as an essential starting point although putting it into context perhaps by using a nursing model for pre-registration or clinical courses may also be desirable. Much of the deliberations of the group will be centred upon the interpretation of the outline syllabus in terms of local conditions and experiences available, nursing systems, preceptor availability on individual units and tutorial expertise may all contribute to final decisions that are made.

An example of a starting point for a content model is given in Figure 11.2 and is the result of a brainstorming session between members of a curriculum planning team. In short, members of this committee envisaged that psychological, biological and sociological aspects as well as health concepts, developmental aspects and professional studies could be taught in relation to activities of living (Roper *et al.*, 1985). Models of nursing, together with their philosophies of intervention or self-care, will be learnt, and as the student progresses, these philosophies will

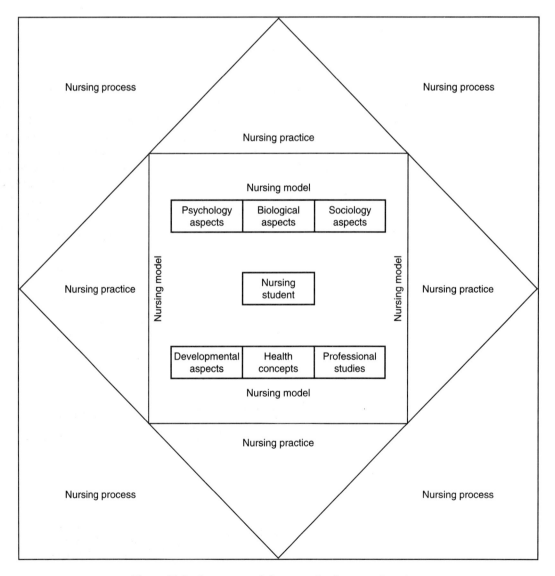

**Figure 11.2.** A conceptual framework of nurse education.

be integrated into their cognitive framework which will enable them to apply their beliefs and knowledge to nursing practice. The nursing process with its assessing, planning and evaluating framework is seen as an organisational structure within which all nursing is learnt and practised.

This is only a very rough draft of a content model and, of course further refinement is necessary. With the above conditions in mind, each subject was then expanded and an example of psychological aspects is given in Figure 11.3.

It can be seen that already decisions are being made regarding the organisation of material in terms of the order in which it is presented. The course content decisions cannot be made in complete isolation from the other components, namely course organisation and learning strategies, although the use of learning outcomes instead of behavioural objectives (see below) will allow the group greater freedom of interpretation of learning experiences as the planning process continues.

## Organisation of course material

Decisions need to be made regarding the organisation of material in order to ensure that learning takes place in a manner which is both acceptable and effective to the student. The availability of experiences in the area, the cost, time constraints, and of course meeting statutory outcomes such as competencies will all guide the group in its discussions.

As well as external influences, decisions regarding the organisation of material will be largely dependent upon the beliefs of the group, particularly in terms of the process *vs* product debate discussed earlier. It may be applicable to utilise an existing curriculum model such as the spiral curriculum (Bruner, 1972), which is essentially a model which allows the building of knowledge through revisiting concepts in an increasingly complex manner throughout the course.

Rolfe (1993) in lucidly describing the spiral curriculum (Figure 11.4) in terms of Kolb's theory

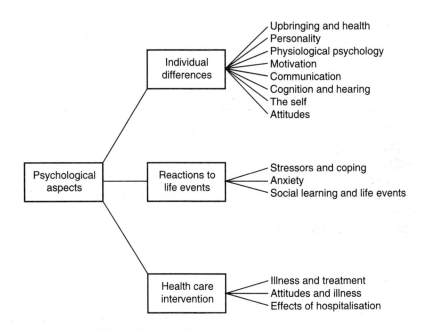

**Figure 11.3.** Psychological aspects of nursing.

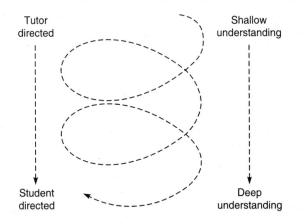

**Figure 11.4** Spiral curriculum (from Rolfe, 1993).

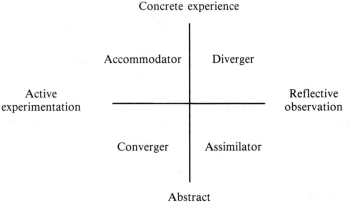

**Figure 11.5** Learning cycle and learning styles (Kolb, 1976).

(Figure 11.5) states that:

Each time the student travels around the cycle from experience to reflection to conceptualisation to experimentation and back to experience he/she does so at a deeper theoretical level and with more control over the process and content.

The use of this sort of curriculum model will, by its very nature, dictate how the experiences will be presented and organised. By using, entirely appropriately, an established learning theory such as Kolb's, statements are being made by the curriculum group about the nature of learning itself. It is an easy mistake to make to consider only the content of the course without taking into account the underlying assumptions about the nature of teaching and learning around which it should take place.

## Learning strategies

Learning strategies need to be considered although it will be apparent to the reader that these may be intrinsically linked to the model chosen for the organisation of material in as far as the model may be humanistic or behaviourally orientated. In any case, the degree to which, for instance, learner autonomy is facilitated will need to be decided within the context of more general deliberations such as meeting national standards. In terms of the spiral curriculum, it may be decided for example, that more teacher-centred strategies will be used at the beginning of the course with more student-centred strategies being introduced as the student gains in knowledge and confidence, in other words when they revisit concepts.

An important point that should be mentioned here is the acceptance of certain strategies by both students and teachers, and indeed preceptors and managers. The merits of a student-centred approach have been mentioned throughout the text, but the practicalities may be quite different. In some studies (e.g. Burnard and Morrison, 1991) it appeared that the favoured teaching strategies of students were teacher centred, and those of teachers, student centred! On the other hand, despite the acceptance of student-centred strategies by teachers, there are still concerns that by using such methods, the curriculum will not be covered (Harris, 1988).

Most of the problems that arise from a new curriculum can be substantially overcome by improving communications with colleagues outside the group at every stage of the curriculum's development and the provision of a comprehensive system of workshops and more formal education before the implementation of the curriculum.

# Assessment

The assessment strategy utilised once again is dependent upon both national and local guidelines. An assessment strategy must be developed alongside the curriculum rather than after it has been written.

# The hidden curriculum

The term *hidden curriculum* refers to those components of the course which are not implicit in the actual document and frequently refers to relationships, social encounters, group activities, etc., which will affect the learning process. The organisation of placements, provision of study time, location of courses, social facilities available, living accommodation, travelling times, as well as personal finances may all help to dictate how effective the student will be in their endeavours.

# Conclusions

Participating in curriculum development from the preceptor's point of view can bring about massive insights into the organisation and structure not only of the whole curriculum but also of the way in which learning can be facilitated effectively in their own area. To be at variance with what has been facilitated in the more formal setting both in terms of content and style has been found to be a major source of anxiety for students.

That participating in such a development can be hard work is not disputed, but if the individual preceptor concerned acts as a representative of their colleagues rather than an autonomous agent, the task may become considerably easier, particularly if a formal group can be set up in the clinical area to aid the process.

Most of all, the fact that both students and preceptors alike are individuals with unique needs may have a bearing when planning a curriculum and assumptions regarding how the individual is to learn can be easily misplaced. There is no substitute for effective communication both in terms of planning and in the execution of the curriculum.

# Summary

Curriculum development is largely governed by the guidelines produced regarding the approvals process, as well as the course development regulations and guidelines.

The course philosophy is developed in line with the philosophy of the college which will normally govern the general conduct of courses, the educational climate and even relationships between students, educationists and managers.

The development of a curriculum ideology must not only be a compilation of the ideas of the whole curriculum team, but should also reflect, through team members, the ideas and beliefs of those whom they represent.

A product-based curriculum relies heavily on behavioural objectives which by their very nature attempt to predict exactly what a student will have learned following an educational experience or course of study.

The process model in its purest form concentrates on the education experience rather than a predictable education outcome and, not surprisingly, relies heavily on the individual learner as the central focus.

The shift towards a process approach appears to be gaining momentum (Crotty, 1993) and this in many ways has to be seen as desirable in as much as it encourages the individual to reach their potential.

The outlining syllabus provided by the awarding authority (National Boards) serve as an essential starting point in curriculum planning.

The availability of experiences in the area, the cost, time constraints, and of course meeting statutory outcomes such as competencies will all guide the group in its discussions.

Most of the problems that arise from a new curriculum can be substantially overcome by improving communications with colleagues outside the group at every stage of the curriculum's development and the provision of a comprehensive system of workshops and more formal education before the implementation of the curriculum.

# Related activities

## Activity 1

1. Identify the different courses, both pre- and post-registration, which are facilitated in your clinical area and select one.
2. Obtain a copy of the philosophy for the course.
3. Obtain a copy of the course curriculum.
4. In approximately 500 words, identify whether the philosophy and the curriculum reflects a product or process approach, or a combination of both, and give reasons for your answer.

## Activity 2

Select a student you are working with

1. Identify between you an area in which they wish to develop during their placement.
2. Agree five learning outcomes between you and a time span of not less than two weeks in which to achieve them.
3. Within the framework of the course philosophy and, if possible, in accordance with the curriculum model, devise a scheme to help the student to achieve these learning outcomes. This may include observation, visits, teaching sessions, practice etc.

# References

Bloom, B.S. (1956) *Taxonomy of Educational Objectives*. Longman.

Bruner, J. (1960) *The Process of Education*. Cambridge, MA: Harvard University Press.

Bruner, J. (1972) *The relevance of education*. London, Allen and Unwin.

Burnard, P. and Morrison, P. (1991) Preferred teaching and learning strategies. *Nursing Times*, **87**(38), 52.

Crotty, M. (1993) Curriculum issues related to the newly developed nursing diploma course. *Nurse Education Today*, **13**, 264–269.

Darbyshire, P. (1991) The American revolution. *Nursing Times*, **87**, 57–58.

ENB (1987) Approval processes for courses in nursing, midwifery and health visiting. Circular 1987/28/MAT.

ENB (1989) Project 2000 – A New Preparation for Practice.

Harris, L. (1988) Student centred learning. *Nursing Times*, **84**(39), 63.

Orem, D. (1985) *Nursing: Concepts of Practice*. New York: McGraw Hill.

Peplau, H. (1952) *Interpersonal Relationships in Nursing*. New York: S P Putman.

Rolfe, G. (1993) Towards a theory of student-centred nurse education: overcoming the constraints of a professional curriculum. *Nurse Education Today*, **13**(2), 149–154.

Roper, N., Logan, W.W. & Tierney (1985) *The Elements of Nursing*, **2nd edn**. Edinburgh: Churchill Livingstone.

Rush, K.L., Ouellet, L.L. and Wasson, D. (1991) Faculty development: the essence of curriculum planning. *Nurse Education Today*, **11**(2), 121–6.

Smith, L. (1987) Application of nursing models to a curriculum: some considerations. *Nurse Education Today*, **7**(3), 109–115.

Stenhouse, L. (1975) *An Introduction to Curriculum Research and Development*. London: Heinemann.

# chapter twelve

# Study skills

## Introduction

The role of communication in teaching and learning has been discussed extensively in Chapter one, but here a more specific discussion on the role of written communication will be entered into. It is difficult, if not impossible, to separate written from verbal communication, and indeed these are usually classed as synonymous in terms of many of the rules that will be applied to them, e.g. the discussion on encoding in Chapter one applies equally to written as well as spoken communication.

With this caution firmly in mind, we will now progress to a more detailed discussion of those areas of written communication most likely to affect the learner and their facilitator. In doing so, it should be remembered that the implications for many of these skills goes far beyond simply essay writing and will obviously have an impact on the everyday management of both the learning environment and the workplace, e.g.

1. Patient assessment.
2. Planning/evaluating care.
3. Writing a report for a new development.
4. Designing an information booklet.
5. Forming the basis for carrying out research.
6. Writing a unit philosophy.
7. Project for a course of study.

## Writing a report

Either as a part of their everyday work or as part of a course of study, nurses are increasingly expected to produce written reports, too frequently without having been taught the skills required. The list above gives just some of the examples where this could happen. In this section we will outline a tried and tested method of producing a report and then give an example of how a report could be written.

## Assessment

1. Identify the reason/need for the report.
2. Where appropriate, discuss with relevant staff first. (It may be necessary to gain their cooperation in implementing any changes.)

## Plan

1. Brainstorm with as many people as necessary to gain ideas about the reports content. A Buzan diagram (Buzan, 1974) has been used in the example to achieve this (see Appendix one).
2. Research the subject. Gain help of the librarian and complete a literature search on the subject. (See Appendix two for details).

## Implementation

Write the report using the following format.

*Title*. The title should say what the report is about. An abstract title simply confuses the reader and decreases the chance of the report being read.

*Introduction*. The introduction should say what the report is about (its content); it should be designed in such a way as to gain the interest and attention of the reader and where appropriate a specific reader that you particularly wish to impress, e.g. the budget holder.

Since many reports develop as they are written, many people write the introduction to a project last. Depending on the size of your report, you should also produce a contents page with page numbers to make it easier for the reader to find their way around the report.

*Main body of the text*. One way to organise this is to use each section of your Buzan diagram as a main heading with the Buzan's subsections as your subheadings (see Appendix one).

When reading through your first draft, check the content for the following:

1. Is the report presented in a clear, logical order with clear headings and subheadings for each section?
2. Is the content unambiguous and easy to understand?
3. Are the spelling and punctuation correct?
4. Have you addressed the reader directly without being condescending or talking over their head? Ensure that specialist terms are always defined clearly.
5. Have you included references to other sections of the project or to other works where appropriate?

## Evaluation

*Conclusions*. (Note that you should never include any new information in this or subsequent parts of the report.)

1. This section should briefly outline the purpose of the report.
2. It is here that you draw your conclusions based on the evidence presented in the report.
3. Your conclusions should be brief and to the point.

## Recommendations

Here you should include your recommendations for changes that may be necessary as a result of your investigations, e.g. change the supplier, implement a new system of interviewing staff, arrange for staff education, etc.

Conclusions and recommendations should be included as one section in short reports.

*References/appendixes*. You should include a list of works referred to in the report using either the Vancouver or Harvard methods of referencing (see Appendix three).

You should also include any questionnaires or other evidence at the end of your report as appendices.

Having completed all of the above content and checks, the next stage is to ask someone to read the report for you to check for the same things. You do not necessarily have to make all of the changes that they ask for but it is a great help to get a fresh view.

Now redraft the report as many times as you feel is necessary until you are completely satisfied that it meets all of the above criteria. Finally you need to consider whether or not you need to ask permission from anyone before you publish. Check to see that you do not contravene the copyright act by using someone else's work without their permission. If you intend to publish the work to a wider audience and you have mentioned your organisation's name, ensure that you get the permission of your line manager before doing so. It is best if this permission is in writing!

## Report example

The report below has been written following the above guidelines. Note that the Buzan diagram (Appendix one) has been used as a format for the report.

# Individualised patient care development on Ward 23

## Introduction

Ward 23, in conjunction with the Education Department, propose to embark on a programme to develop a system of individualised patient care. The programme follows a pattern that has been tried and tested in other hospitals and should result in a unique adapted nursing model based on the ward's philosophy of care.

This development is proposed following the recent educational audit which states that if Ward 23 is to continue to provide student nurses with experience, the individualised patient care system in operation must be updated.

It is intended to form a facilitators group which will lead the ward team in the following developments:

1. Write a ward philosophy of care.
2. Select a nursing model based on that philosophy.
3. Adapt the model to meet the ward's special requirements.
4. Organise the education of other ward staff members.
5. Design the documentation in accordance with "3" above.
6. Run a pilot study to identify positive and negative aspects of the system.
7. Make changes that are necessary and continue to run pilot studies until all ward staff members are happy with the new system.

# 1. Facilitators group

A two-day programme will be run by the education department (based on the Open University Programme "A Systematic Approach to Nursing Care") to prepare up to six members of nursing staff from Ward 23 to lead the developments taking place. This group will be known as Development Facilitators and will be made up of staff from day and night duty to ensure involvement of the total ward team.

Discussions have already taken place with the ward teacher who has agreed to run this two-day programme.

The programme will explore the following topics:

1. Philosophy of nursing.
2. Nursing models (Orem and Roper).
3. Nursing diagnosis.
4. Assessment/planning/evaluation.
5. Primary nursing.
6. Accountability in nursing.
7. Educational resources.

The facilitators group will then meet once every three weeks at 1400 to control each stage of the development. This group will be responsible for leading the ward team in each stage of the development as outlined in the introduction above. They will also be responsible for the liaison with other ward staff and any education and support that will be necessary to ensure that all staff are familiar with the development at each stage. The involvement and cooperation of all staff at each stage is seen as crucial to the success of the development.

# 2. Writing the ward Statement of Beliefs

The first step in the developments described above is to write the ward's Statement of Nursing Beliefs. Each individual involved in nursing care will be asked to write their own personal beliefs about nursing. A sheet designed for this purpose will be provided (see appendix). In addition to nursing staff, 10 patients and all medical staff attending the ward will be asked to complete this form.

In order for the programme to move ahead at a reasonable pace, a two-week deadline will be put on this exercise.

The individual ideas will then be put together into one document. This document, in the form of a questionnaire, will be given to each member of staff who will be asked to comment about each statement, e.g. whether they approve or not. As a result of this survey, the Ward 23 Statement of Beliefs will be produced.

This Statement of Beliefs will guide the choice of nursing model and its eventual adaptation. It is important therefore that everyone has a say and that it is truly the beliefs of all staff.

# 3. Selection and adaptation of the nursing model

The facilitators group will then select a nursing model based on the beliefs of the nursing staff. If, for example, the staff emphasise the importance of patient involvement in their own care, it may be appropriate to select the Orem Model (Walsh, 1991). The group may decide, on the other hand that a combination of two models such as Orem and Roper may be more appropriate.

Having made their selection, the group will design the assessment tool, care plan and evaluation sheet. The views of the whole nursing team will be ascertained at each stage of the development to ensure cooperation and validity. The education department and nursing management will also be asked to comment to ensure accuracy and the legality of the documents.

## 4. Short pilot study

A small group of patients which reflects the general work of the ward will be selected and the documents will be tested over a period of two weeks. All ward staff will be involved in this pilot study to ensure that they understand the development as it takes place and can make their comments for inclusion in any changes that may take place as a result.

The documentation will be adapted as a result of comments from nursing staff, education staff and nursing management, and if necessary, other similar pilot studies will be run until staff are reasonably happy that the tool will work for their group of patients.

## 5. Long pilot study

The documentation at this stage will be printed and a pilot study lasting six months will take place using all patients admitted to Ward 23. At the end of this period, all staff will be completely familiar with the system and any final changes can be made.

## 6. Conclusion and recommendation

It can be seen that if Ward 23 wish to continue to provide experience for student nurses that this development is essential. The College of Nursing will remove students from the ward unless it can be demonstrated that this has occurred before the next educational audit in 12 months time. The development will also afford the trained staff with the opportunity to look critically at their practice and continue its development in the light of current nursing research. The development will benefit patients and their relatives by improving communications, continuity of care and where appropriate, direct involvement in their own care.

It is therefore recommended that the development commence as soon as possible.

Sister Care (Ward 23)

## Appendix

### Individual statements of beliefs about nursing

Every nurse develops his/her own beliefs about nursing based on a wide range of knowledge and experience over a period of years. While it is not something that we think about on a day-to-day basis, our beliefs govern everything that we do in nursing as well as our lives in general. A ward Statement of Beliefs should reflect the beliefs of all that work in that ward if it is to be used to decide the way care is organised. Therefore, everyone involved in the provision of nursing care on Ward 23 has been asked to write their own individual Statement of Beliefs.

To complete this exercise, simply write short statements on the attached sheet that reflect what you believe to be true about the provision of nursing care. For example,

1. I believe that all patients have the right to take part in the decisions that are made about their treatment and nursing care.
2. I believe that the patient should be treated as an individual and that their individual needs should be considered in the provision of all nursing care.

Please complete your Statement of Belief about nursing below and return to Sister Care by: ..................
Thank you for taking part in this exercise.

1.

2.

3.

4.

5.

6.

7.

8.

Please continue overleaf!

## Bibliography

Akinsanya, J.A. (1989) *Recent Advances in Nursing Theories and Models of Nursing*. London: Churchill Livingstone.
Cormack (1984) *The Research Process in Nursing*. London: Blackwell Scientific.
Fitzpatrick, J. and Whall, A. (1983) *Conceptual Models of Nursing*. New York: Brady.
Kershaw, B. and Salvage, J. (1986) *Models for Nursing*. Chichester: John Wiley and Sons.
Orem, D.E. (1985) *Nursing. Concepts of Practice*. New York, McGraw Hill.
Roper, N., Logan, W.W. and Tierney, A.J. (1980) *The Elements of Nursing*. London: Churchill Livingstone.
Walsh, M. (1991) *Models in Clinical Nursing*. London: Baillière Tindall.
Wright, S. (1986) *Building and Using a Model of Nursing*. London: Edward Arnold.

Please note that information such as cost of the development and educational resources has not been included. An actual report may need to include more information but the format will remain the same.

## Reading skills

When studying any subject, there are usually a very large number of texts, journal articles and other references to choose from. Even with good advice about the most useful sources of information, this can still be a daunting task. It is of the utmost importance therefore that the time spent reading is used to the best possible effect.

A common problem that many people experience is that of concentrating for any extended period of time. This is due in part to the fact that our reading is not organised. It is difficult to concentrate if specific goals have not been set at the outset.

The SQ3R method described below can help to overcome this problem for the busy practitioner and is a method that can easily be taught to students to help them make more effective use of their reading time.

### SQ3R

To Survey, Question, Read, Recite and Review, or SQ3R (Beard, 1987) is a way of organising reading in a systematic and methodical manner which helps the reader not only to concentrate for longer periods of time, but also improves the quality and relevance of the information that is gained from the exercise. At the end of an hour spent reading, you should be able to state clearly what you have gained, have a record that can be used for future reference or revision and have a clearer idea of how to approach this subject in the future.

Having read the following description, try the Activity 2 at the end of the chapter to see if this method could improve your own reading skills and that of your students.

## Survey

The purpose of making a survey of the text is to avoid wasting valuable time reading material not relevant. It asks the question, "What is this text about?". You can find this out in the following way:

1. Read the contents page to identify any specific chapters related to your subject.
2. Read the preface or foreword. This is written by the author to let the reader know what the book is about and may give specific information about the book such as the audience it was written for, and any special features of the format, such as exercises.
3. Look at the index to identify other chapters which may contain relevant information.
4. Look briefly at one or two chapters to familiarise yourself with the format being used.

This process will only take you a short time, and at the end of it, you should be absolutely clear about whether this book is suitable for the task you have to complete.

## Question

Write down a list of questions on a sheet of paper and then ask yourself "Where in the text will I find the answers?". The time spent in surveying the book will help with this but you also need to go further to find the answers.

## Read

Having found the relevant chapter(s) in the book, read through the information carefully. While reading, you should actively search for the answers to the questions set earlier. Depending on the degree of difficulty, it may be necessary to read the text several times and make notes for future use.

Once the "read" stage has been completed you should wait for at least 24 hours before going on to the "recite" stage of this process.

## Recite

The purpose of this stage is to ask the question, "What has been learned about this subject?". This can be done alone, but best results are achieved if completed with at least one other person. Explain to another student or your course tutor, in your own words and without the use of notes, what you understand about the subject. In this way it will become clear whether you understand the subject or not and may provide guidance for any further reading that may be necessary.

*Review*

At this point, it is worth reviewing the process that has occurred. Ask yourself the following questions:

1. Is my knowledge on this subject sufficient?
2. Where do I go from here?
3. What further information do I require?
4. Which other sources of information are available?

In answering these four questions, the student will ensure that the learning process is accurate and relevant. This is a form of self-assessment which will not only result in an improvement in knowledge level but also improve the skill of using the SQ3R method.

When the student has practised the SQ3R method and is quite confident, it is worth considering how it could be adapted to suit the individual and the subject being studied. The process will be even more successful when adapted in this way.

# Summary

It is difficult, if not impossible to separate written from verbal communication and indeed these are usually classed as synonymous.

Nurses are increasingly expected to produce written reports, too frequently without having been taught the skills required.

Guidelines for *writing a report*:

1. Assessment − reason/need for the report.
2. *Plan* − Buzan diagram, research.
3. *Implementation* − title, introduction, main body of text.
4. *Evaluation* − conclusions, recommendations, references and appendixes.

To Survey, Question, Read, Recite and Review, or SQ3R (Beard, 1992) is a way of organising reading in a systematic and methodical manner which helps the reader not only to concentrate for longer periods of time, but also improves the quality and relevance of the information that is gained from the exercise.

# Related activities

## Activity 1

Produce a short report, following the guidelines below, which describes the necessity for trained nurses to keep up to date, including proposals for how that can be achieved:

1. Produce a Buzan diagram (see Appendix one).
2. Search the literature (see Appendix two).
3. Write your report including:
   (a) Title (central theme from the Buzan diagram).
   (b) Introduction.
   (c) Development (using subheadings from the Buzan diagram).

(d) Conclusions and recommendations combined.
(e) Appendixes.
(f) References (see Appendix three).
4. Present your report to your nurse manager.

## Activity 2

Before deciding whether you would use the SQ3R method or would teach it to a student, try the following exercise. You should aim to complete it in approximately one hour.

Answer the following, using the SQ3R method:

How would you assess a patient using the Roper model of nursing?

Example text:

Walsh, M (1991) *Models in Clinical Nursing: the Way Forward*. London: Baillière Tindall.

If preferred, select a subject that you are working on at the moment and a reference relevant to that subject.

When you are sure that you understand the process, teach one student how to use the SQ3R method.

# References

Beard, R. (1992) SQ3R. In G.J. Fairbairne and C. Winch (eds) *Reading Writing and Reasoning*. Milton Keynes: Open University Press.

Binnie A., Bond, S., Law, G. *et al*. (1991) *A Systematic Approach to Nursing Care: An Introduction*. Milton Keynes: Open University Press.

Buzan, T. (1974) *Use Your Head*. BBC Publications.

Walsh, M. (1991) *Models in Clinical Nursing: the Way Forward*. London: Baillière Tindall.

# appendix one

# Designing a Buzan diagram

A Buzan diagram can be used as a method of constructing knowledge patterns (Buzan, 1974) or, as in this case, of brainstorming a subject to form the basis for writing a report. As seen in Figure A1.1 the idea is to have the main theme at the centre with related subjects branching out. Each branch can then be further developed with sub-branches and so on. Links can be made between the branches and sub-branches where appropriate. This can be produced by an individual or group based solely on their existing knowledge and then built upon when the literature search has been completed. It may well form the basis for the literature search. It is further suggested that the diagram could be used to construct the report with the main theme at the centre forming the title, the branches forming headings and sub-branches forming the subheadings in the report.

## Activity

Buzan diagrams or concept maps are a very useful way of clarifying your thoughts about a given subject. Produce one for yourself and see how quickly you can develop a subject of your choice.

The following should be included:

1. Select a topic.
2. Write the main theme at the centre of a sheet of A4 paper.
3. Identify at least six topics which relate to the main theme and write them on your sheet around the centre. These should be joined to the central theme with a straight line. Ensure that enough space is left for subheadings.
4. Think of at least two subheadings for each of the topics in "3" above and include these on the sheet.
5. Look at the finished diagram and identify any links between the headings and subheadings, other than to the central theme. Show these links by drawing a line between the two.

Finally, explain the above process to a student nurse and help them to develop their own concept map. Ensure that they understand the process by reading through their finished product and make any useful suggestions necessary.

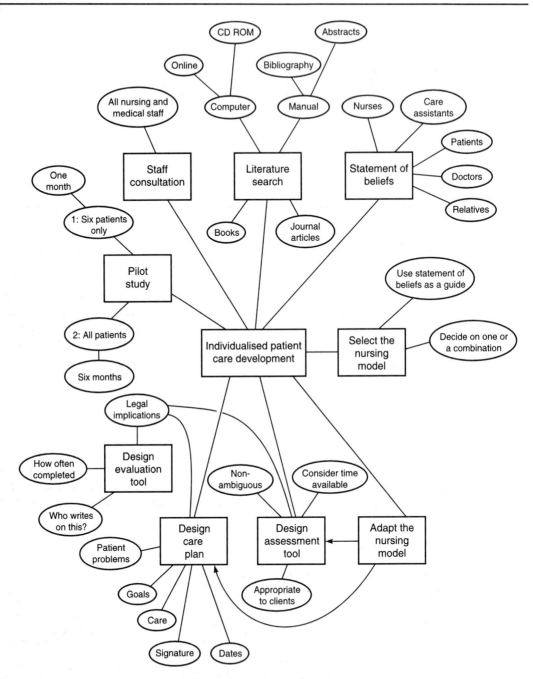

**Figure A1.1.** Buzan diagram.

# appendix two

# Searching the literature

Completing a literature search for the first time can be a very daunting task indeed. There are so many different tools available to you that most people are unsure about where to begin. Fear not, help is always at hand in the form of the librarian. This person is the expert, and even experienced researchers will ask their advice before starting. The purpose of this exercise is for you to gain a good knowledge of your subject by reading the published material available. You may also identify tools such as questionnaires that have been previously validated and could be used directly or adapted for use in your own development. Note that you will need to get permission from the author in this case.

## Books

All libraries will have an author catalogue and subject catalogue available. Some will have their book stock on a computer data base which makes the search quicker and easier once you understand how the system works. The books on your particular subject will be a valuable source of background material and, if recently published, references for further reading.

## Journals

You could start by carrying out a manual search of the journals by using the various abstracts and indices available. These are publications which list subjects in journal articles in alphabetical order; each one is slightly different, so ask the librarian if you are unsure. Examples of these are *The Nursing Research Abstracts*, *RCN Bibliography*, *Health Service Abstracts* and *ASSIA*. You can complete quite a comprehensive literature search using this type of publication. The advantage of doing a manual search is that while browsing through these references, you will always find many others that you were not looking for but that are relevant to your subject.

A similar search can be carried out using a computer either by "on-line searching" or using "CD ROM". On-line searching is where one computer searches the data base of another computer via a telephone link. The CD ROM is a compact disc, on to which the data base is updated at regular intervals through the year, and can be searched in the library itself.

A word of caution about computer searches: unless the search is designed very carefully, you will find that you will have all sorts of irrelevant material printed out, and considering you will have to pay for each search, this can be very costly. The librarian will help here too! Always ask for advice.

# Activity

It is essential for any teacher to have a good working knowledge of the library used by the group of students they come into contact with. This exercise is designed to help the teacher familiarise themselves with their nursing library and to sharpen their library skills so that they are in a better position to advise students in their study.

1. Choose a subject that you need to find information about, possibly related to a teaching session that is being planned.
2. Using the following methods, carry out a search of the books available:
   (a) Using the subject index and the author index, carry out a manual search of your chosen subject.
   (b) The library may have their book stocks listed on computer. If this is the case ask the librarian to show you how the system works and carry out a search. Now that you are familiar with the relevant books available, write a list of at least three references using the Harvard method and three references using the Vancouver method of referencing (Appendix three).
3. Now carry out a search of the relevant journals:
   (a) You will find the journal stock in the reference section of the library. The current additions should be on a rack. Familiarise yourself with these, noting any specialist journals relating to your subject.
   (b) Ask the librarian which abstracts and indexes are available, e.g. *RCN Bibliography*, *NHS Abstracts*, *Research Abstracts*.
   (c) Select one of these and make a search to find journal articles on your chosen subject. Use the most recent copies of the abstract or index to find at least six articles. (This should include at least two pieces of research.)
   (d) Using the references from (c), find the articles from the back copies of journals kept on the library shelves. You may wish to photocopy some of these for later use if they are of particular value.
   Write out three of the references using the Harvard method and three using the Vancouver method (Appendix three).

For those who previously were not familiar with their own nursing library, this exercise will show you how quick and easy it is to find up to date information which can be used to teach students and may be used to update nursing practices. Always remember, that if you have any difficulties, ask the librarian for help, he/she is the expert.

# appendix three

# Writing references

## Harvard style

In this style the references are listed in alphabetical order. In the text, the reference is identified by the name of the author and the date of the work given in brackets. Two articles by the same author in the same year are distinguished by letters, "a" for the first, "b" for the second and so on.

The details that should appear in the reference list are as follows.

### Journal articles

Author(s), (year of publication in brackets), article title, journal title, volume number (part number in brackets), page number(s).

Example:

Vin Tsu Vyuyan, M. (1992) Making Sense of Hypothermia. Nursing Times, 88(49), 38–40.

### Complete textbook

Author(s), (year of publication in brackets), book title including edition if not first edition, place of publication, publisher's name.

Example:

Oliver, R. (1993) Psychology and Health Care. London: Baillière Tindall.

### Chapter in textbook

Author(s) of chapter (year of publication in brackets), title of chapter, in, author(s)/editor(s) of complete work, title of complete work, including edition if not first edition, place of publication, publisher's name.

Example:

Yeats, J. (1990) Respecting clients' dignity. In: Professional Nurse, The Ward Sister's Survival Guide. London: Austen Cornish.

# Vancouver style

This style is used in *Index Medicus* and several of the major publishers are endeavouring to standardise on this. This style uses a system of sequential numbering; each reference is cited in the text using a number, either in square brackets, or set superior to the line, i.e. the first citation would be "[1]" or "[1]", the next "[2]" or "[2]" and so on. The list of references at the end of the article should appear in this numerical order.

The details in the reference list should be arranged as follows.

## *Journal articles*

Author(s), article title, journal title, year of publication, volume number (part number in brackets), page number(s).

Example:

1. Yin Tsu Vyuyan M. Making sense of hypothermia. Nursing Times 1992; 88(49): 38-40.

## *Complete textbook*

Author(s), book title including edition if not first edition, place of publication, publisher's name, year of publication.

Example:

2. Oliver R. Psychology and Health Care, London, Baillière Tindall, 1993.

## *Chapter in textbook*

Author(s) of chapter, title of chapter including edition if not first edition, in, author(s)/editor(s) of complete work, title of complete work, place of publication, publisher's name, year of publication.

Example:

3. Yeats J. Respecting clients' dignity, in Professional Nurse, The Ward Sister's Survival Guide, London, Austen Cornish, 1990.

If the publication was written by more than three authors, the first three names only are quoted, followed by the abbreviation "*et al.*".

Never cite a publication appearing in someone else's list of references without actually reading it. It could differ greatly in content from that which is implied in their work, and the reference could even be wrongly cited!

# Nurses, midwives and health visitors (training) amendment rules, 1989

## The nurses midwives & health visitors act 1979

*Rule 18A*

1. The content of the Common Foundation Programme and the Branch Programme shall be such as the Council may from time to time require.
2. The Common Foundation Programme and the Branch programme shall be designed to prepare the student to assume the responsibilities and accountability that registration confers, and to prepare the nursing student to apply knowledge and skills to meet the nursing needs of individuals and of groups in health and in sickness in the area of practice of the Branch Programme, and shall include enabling the student to achieve the following outcomes:
   (a) the identification of the social and health implications of pregnancy and child bearing, physical and mental handicap, disease, disability, or ageing for the individual, her or his friends, family and community;
   (b) the recognition of common factors which contribute to, and those which adversely affect, physical, mental and social well-being of patients and clients and take appropriate action;
   (c) the use of relevant literature and research to inform the practice of nursing;
   (d) the appreciation of the influence of social, political and cultural factors in relation to health care;
   (e) an understanding of the requirements of legislation relevant to the practice of nursing;
   (f) the use of appropriate communication skills to enable the development of helpful, caring relationships with patients and clients and their families and friends, and to initiate and conduct therapeutic relationships with patients and clients;
   (g) the identification of health related learning needs of patients and clients, families and friends and to participate in health promotion;

(h) an understanding of the ethics of health care and of the nursing profession and the responsibilities which these impose on the nurse's professional practice;

(i) the identification of the needs of patients and clients to enable them to progress from varying degrees of dependence to maximum independence, or to a peaceful death;

(j) the identification of physical, psychological, social and spiritual needs of the patient or client; an awareness of values and concepts of individual care; the ability to devise a plan of care, contribute to its implementation and evaluation; and the demonstration of the application of the principles of a problem-solving approach to the practice of nursing;

(k) the ability to function effectively in a team and participate in a multi-professional approach to the care of patients and clients;

(l) the use of the appropriate channel of referral for matters not within her sphere of competence;

(m) the assignment of appropriate duties to others and the supervision, teaching and monitoring of assigned duties.

# Glossary

**Accommodators**  Those with strong concrete experience and active experimentation skills.

**Acoustic code**  In terms of memory, information which is represented as auditory features. Also called phonemic code.

**Advanced organiser**  In reception learning (Ausubel; see Chapter 5), introductory material that is presented ahead of the learning task and at a higher level of abstraction and inclusiveness than the learning task itself.

**Adaptors**  Attempts to maintain self-control, e.g. fidgeting.

**Affect displays**  The expression of emotion, e.g by facial expression.

**Altruism**  Rendering help to other persons without thought of personal gain or reward.

**Amygdala**  Brain structure thought to be involved in the consolidation of new memories. Located below the cerebral cortex.

**Articulatory loop**  In the "working memory model", it holds the words we are about to say, and also acts as a rehearsal loop. It is used whenever we verbally repeat material in order to memorise it. It therefore deals with the articulation of verbal material and is considered as an "inner voice".

**Assimilators**  Those with highly developed abstract conceptualisation and reflective observation competencies.

**Attitude**  A mental and neural state of readiness, organised through experience, exerting a directive or dynamic influence upon the individual's response to all objects and situations with which it is related.

**Baton sign**  Hand gestures.

**Behavioural objective**  A learning objective where the outcome of learning is directly observable and, to a large extent, predictable.

**Central Executive**  In the working memory model, the central executive stores information for short periods of time, can process information from sensory inputs in a variety of ways and is involved in tasks such as reading writing, problem solving, mental arithmetic and learning.

**Classical conditioning**  Originally described by Pavlov, the theory is concerned with reflexes, and attributes all learning to conditioning. Alternatively it can be described as responses to specific stimuli.

**Closure**  In Gestalt psychology, the grouping together of elements of a figure or, for instance, learning material, so as to complete the picture or subject.

**Cognitive dissonance**  Cognitions regarding a situation or behaviour that are mutually exclusive.

**Conditional positive regard**  When significant others only value the individual when their behaviour is seen as correct.

**Conditioned reflexes**  In classical conditioning, reflexes formed as a result of experience.

**Conditioned stimulus**  In classical conditioning, a previously neutral item which, through "pairing" with an unconditioned stimulus, produces a new response.

**Conditions of worth**  The standards that the individual perceives they must attain in order to receive conditional positive regard from others (Rogers; see Chapter 5).

**Convergent Assessment**   Typically a final standard examination which tells the assessor more about the similarities between students rather than the ways in which they diverge. Certain project work could be said to be divergent but only if the individual is allowed to explore and investigate in an individual manner.

**Convergers**   Those with strong abstract conceptualisation and active experimentation skills.

**Decoding**   The process by which we translate words back into ideas.

**Discovery learning**   Learning which places emphasis on learner-centred approaches, valued first-hand experience, experimentation and the development of critical abilities.

**Divergent assessment**   Assessment that examines the individual's development in contrast to the convergent assessment (typically a final standard examination) which tells the assessor more about the similarities between students rather than the ways in which they diverge.

**Divergers**   Those with strong concrete experience and reflective observation skills.

**Ego state**   System of feelings accompanied by a set of coherent behaviour patterns.

**Elaborate code**   A message which is imparted with detail as distinct from just a statement or command.

**Emblems**   Signs which are complete in themselves, such as the "thumbs-up" sign.

**Emotional dependency**   Seeking help in order to gain praise and attention.

**Encoding**   The process of converting an idea into symbols (words).

**Errorful learning**   In discovery learning, trial and error strategies in which there is a high probability of errors and mistakes before an acceptable generalisation is possible.

**Formative Assessment**   Refers to the process of assertaining a students progress during a course of study or experience in, usually, an informal way. It is usually individually based and will not normally be counted towards a final mark or grade **Gestalt Psychology** School of Psychology which studies perception in terms of inherent organisation and patterns.

**Group climate**   A global way of characterising the structural properties of the group.

**Hidden curriculum**   Those components of the course which are not implicit in the actual document.

**Humanistic psychology**   An approach to psychology based on the subjective experiences and values of the individual, that emphasises the uniqueness of human beings.

**Idiographic assessment**   Assessment that attempts to discover the uniqueness of the individual.

**Illustrators**   Signs which supplement speech, e.g. pointing whilst giving directions.

**Instrumental dependency**   A means for the individual to attain something (such as comfort, relief from physical illness and sometimes building of self-esteem) which may not be achieved independently for one reason or another.

**Law of Pragnanz**   The basic principle that suggests that the perceptual response in any given situation will be the most economical one possible.

**Learning outcome**   Identification of situations in which the individual will participate and serves as a theme around which skills and understandings can be brought to bear in an individual way.

**Mentor**   A person selected by the student to assist, befriend, guide, advise and counsel (but who would not normally be involved in the formal supervision or assessment of that particular student).

**Noise**   Interference with the communication process.

**Nomothetic assessments**   Concerned with a more standardised form of data collection from the process (marking, streaming, etc.).

**Non-verbal leakage**   The process of physical responses which are conveying a different message to the words being used at the time.

**Operant conditioning**   Also known as Type 2 conditioning. Behaviour which is governed by the degree and direction of reinforcement given (Skinner; see Chapter 5).

**Outcome criteria** Relate to the desired effect of, e.g. education in terms of student behaviours, responses, level of knowledge and application of that knowledge.

**Portfolio** Predominantly student-centred, and largely self-assessed in a formative sense. A portfolio can be loosely described as a collection of varied materials such as journals which by definition will include the individual's reflections, profiles, project work, results of peer- and self-assessments.

**Positive regard** Warmth, liking, respect, sympathy and acceptance from another person.

**Positive self-regard** Liking and accepting oneself in the absence of specific contacts with others. A learned human need, derived from the need for positive regard (Rogers; see Chapter 5).

**Preceptor** A combination of the roles of mentor, supervisor and assessor.

**Prejudice** An antipathy based on a faulty and inflexible generalisation directed towards a group as a whole or towards an individual because they are a member of that group.

**Primary acoustic store** In the "working memory model", the primary acoustic store is dependent upon the articulatory loop for the translation of visual information in an acoustic code, but deals with auditory information directly. This store can be used when reading and the printed matter can be "heard" as we read. This store can be referred to as the "inner ear".

**Process assessment** Carried out through techniques such as projects, student-centred learning and contract learning, its purpose is to reveal how a student has learned where as product will merely reveal the end result of the process.

**Process criteria** Relate to actions undertaken by tutorial staff in conjunction with students, service managers, etc.

**Profiles** Multidimensional methods of presenting information usually about individuals and their achievements, attributes or performances

**Progressive differentiation** In reception learning (Ausubel; see Chapter 5) it is the presentation of general ideas first (advanced organisers) followed by gradual increase in details and specificity.

**Quality assurance** The measurement of the actual level of the service provided plus the efforts to modify when necessary the provision of these services in the light of the results of these measurements.

**Restricted Code** A message given without detail and with minimal or no explanation. Usually just a statement or command.

**Self-actualisation** In humanistic psychology, the individuals striving towards their maximum potential.

**Sociogram** A diagrammatic representation of the interrelationships within a group.

**Sociometry** A technique for identifying the structure of groups in terms of the nature of relationships between its members.

**Standard** Professionally agreed level of performance for a particular population which is achievable, observable, desirable and measurable.

**Standard statement** A statement which describes the broad objectives of a standard.

**Structure criteria** Relate to resources in the system which are necessary for the successful completion of the task/area under review.

**Summative assessment** The assessing of learning which has taken place and hopefully applied to practice and is most obviously typified by a final examination which is usually written.

**Transactional analysis** The diagnosis of which ego state implemented a transactional stimulus and which one executed the transactional response.

**Unconditional positive self-regard** A utopian state of complete self-acceptance, free from any conditions of worth (Rogers).

**Unconditioned reflex** In classical conditioning theory, the normal to an unconditioned stimulus such as food.

**Validity**  An examination of the approximate truth or falsity of the propositions.

**Values**  Beliefs that something is good and desirable.

**Visual–spatial scratch pad**  In the "working memory model", this is responsible for dealing with visual and spatial information. It has a limited capacity, and utilises rehearsal. It can be regarded as the "inner eye".

# Index